Coeliac Disease

Alex Gazzola is a health journalist
hundred publications in twenty countr
including *Living with Food Intolerance,*
and has a special interest in food sensi…
disease, about which he writes and blogs regularly. His website is at
<www.alexgazzola.co.uk>.

D0537928

Overcoming Common Problems Series

Selected titles

A full list of titles is available from Sheldon Press,
36 Causton Street, London SW1P 4ST and on our website at
www.sheldonpress.co.uk

Overcoming Common Problems

Coeliac Disease

What you need to know

ALEX GAZZOLA

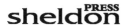

First published in Great Britain in 2011

Sheldon Press
36 Causton Street
London SW1P 4ST
www.sheldonpress.co.uk

British Library Cataloguing-in-Publication Data
A catalogue record for this book is available from the British Library

ISBN 978-1-84709-131-4

1 3 5 7 9 10 8 6 4 2

Typeset by Fakenham Prepress Solutions, Fakenham, Norfolk NR21 8NN
Printed in Great Britain by Ashford Colour Press

Produced on paper from sustainable forests

Contents

Foreword by Dr Chris Steele

Long before I was diagnosed with coeliac disease and even before I became the resident doctor on ITV's *This Morning*, I was particularly concerned with health issues which had a big impact on people's lives but weren't well known. I feel that it is my duty as a general practitioner to get to the root of people's problems and begin the process of healing, even though at times diagnosis and treatment can be complicated processes. This is why the widespread misunderstanding and confusion surrounding coeliac disease sparked such an interest in me.

I was appointed Health Ambassador for Coeliac UK in July 2007, just months before I received the MBE from Her Majesty the Queen, and relished the opportunity to work alongside a national charity doing such great work to support people with the condition and in raising awareness. Once I had learned more about its work I was keen to get involved and I haven't looked back since.

My position as Coeliac UK's Health Ambassador began to make clear to me the level of suffering that some people endure until they get an accurate diagnosis. I had never considered that the condition would have such a direct effect on my own life.

When I became ill it seemed impossible to me that the symptoms I was experiencing could be coeliac disease. As a doctor it is difficult to interpret your own symptoms objectively, so I became another coeliac who was misdiagnosed with irritable bowel syndrome (IBS). I was losing weight rapidly and was regularly gripped with terrible stomach pains and troublesome diarrhoea. Despite treatment for IBS my symptoms persisted so I returned to my gastroenterologist who performed a blood test and intestinal biopsy for coeliac disease. The disturbing factor for me was the not knowing – and although the positive diagnosis came as a shock, I was grateful to have answers.

My diagnosis reinforces my drive to raise awareness of coeliac disease and illustrates the importance of quick and accurate recognition of the condition. My work with Coeliac UK has been incredibly rewarding, and I have seen real growth in awareness of the condition, something to which I think *Coeliac Disease: What you need to know* will contribute.

Now that I am on a strict gluten-free diet for life, I realize how difficult it can sometimes be to stick to this, the only treatment for coeliac disease, and maintain the lifestyle I was used to. Even in the short time I've been diagnosed I've seen an improvement in restaurants and shops selling gluten-free food, but this does need to get better so that we can eat out without the worry.

One of the reasons I struggled to identify my own coeliac disease was the wide-ranging list of complaints that can be associated with it. Alex Gazzola's book addresses this by comprehensively listing the full spectrum of symptoms associated with coeliac disease in a step-by-step introduction to the condition as a whole.

To the casual reader, this book will be impressive because of the amount of interesting information available. To those who have coeliac disease it will provide a lifeline which allows them to allay their own fears while learning of the advances in medical research and the food industry in recent years. Diagnosis is the first challenge. There are half a million people living with symptoms in the UK who have not been diagnosed and are not even aware of how much better they could feel on a gluten-free diet.

It was a great honour to be asked to write the foreword to such a thorough look into the world of this condition. Coeliac disease represents a confusing journey for so many people, and this book provides an accurate and supportive guide to help clear away the fog along the way.

Dr Chris Steele MBE
ITV *This Morning*
Health Ambassador, Coeliac UK

Acknowledgements

I am grateful to all those with coeliac disease or working with those with coeliac disease who have spoken to me about the condition since I started writing about it in 2004, and whose knowledge of and expertise in this fascinating illness has found its way in some form or other into this book. In particular, I'd like to thank Susan Cane, Dr William Dickey, Professor Alessio Fasano, Professor David Sanders – and Norma McGough, Kate Newman, Amy Peterson, Dr Chris Steele and all at Coeliac UK.

In addition, thanks to Michelle Berriedale-Johnson, Fiona Marshall and Eve Menezes Cunningham.

On a personal note, thanks and love to F, R and S.

Introduction

Coeliac disease hasn't always been with us because gluten hasn't always been with us.

For most of the 200,000 years during which we humans have been around to nourish ourselves, we've done so by foraging for vegetables, roots, fruits, nuts, leaves, grubs and insects – supplemented with the odd feast of scavenged or hunted meat.

Around 10,000 years ago, we observed that the watered seeds of plants could give life to new plants of the same kind, which in turn would grow, eventually to bear more seeds. From there, the leap to cultivating plant-based crops and building permanent bases around these new sources of food was a swift one. The hunter-gatherer lifestyle gave way to one of agriculture and settlement. The Neolithic agricultural revolution had begun.

Barley and ancient forms of wheat – einkorn, emmer – were cultivated first in the Fertile Crescent, and later more widely, as our ancestors migrated from the Middle East to China, Europe and beyond. The domestication of animals introduced their protein-rich products – milk, eggs – into our diets too. These were all novel foods to humans. Never underestimate the human capacity to adapt – it is why we are still flourishing – but not everyone's bodies could manage the transition so seamlessly. Food sensitivities began to emerge.

These intolerances are unlikely to have been considered new illnesses. Coeliac disease would have been looked upon much as any other severe, unpleasant disease characterized by the not unfamiliar symptoms of diarrhoea, wasting and general malaise common at the time, due to any number of bacterial infections and gastrointestinal upsets that would routinely have shortened lives. We must assume deaths related to coeliac disease – especially in the young – continued grimly for many years.

It was a Greek physician, Aretaeus of Cappodocia, who first distinguished – and named – coeliac disease in the first century AD. 'If the stomach be irretentive of the food and if it pass through undigested and crude, and nothing ascends into the body, we call such persons coeliacs,' he was found to have written, when his medical texts were translated into English in the nineteenth century. (The word 'coeliac' was derived from Aretaeus' use of the Greek word *koiliakós*, meaning 'suffering in the bowels'.) It is remarkable how astutely he recognized the poor absorption of nutrition that characterizes classical coeliac disease.

Aretaeus had also observed that 'bread is rarely suitable for giving strength', but little progress was made on the dietary connection until Dr Matthew Baillie, an early nineteenth-century physician, noted that some of his coeliac patients 'have appeared to derive considerable advantage from living almost entirely upon rice'. Yet even this observation was largely overlooked, and it wasn't until the late nineteenth century that paediatrician Samuel Gee, renowned lecturer in medicine at St Bart's Hospital, London, moved us a step forward.

'A kind of chronic indigestion which is met with in persons of all ages,' was how Gee described the illness he dubbed the coeliac 'affection'. He wrote of the 'wasting, weakness and pallor' of patients and noted rightly that 'if the patient can be cured at all, it must be by means of diet'. He was almost there when he stated that 'the allowance of farinaceous [floury] food must be small', yet his diets were imperfect: they recommended meats and mussels but also thin slices of toast, and they disallowed fruit, vegetables and safe sources of starchy carbohydrate. There would have been improvements on such a lower-gluten diet, but not relief by any means.

Progress was patchy in subsequent decades. It was observed that non-diarrhoeal forms of coeliac disease could exist, and that there was a greater co-incidence among family members.

In 1924 the banana diet became popular. Introduced by American paediatrician Sidney Haas, who attempted it experimentally on several children whose health subsequently improved, the diet eliminated potatoes, breads and all cereals, and remained the treatment of choice for several decades, doubtlessly sparing lives. Haas believed it was the removal of carbohydrate that drove recuperation in coeliac patients, and he maintained this conviction long after it had been demonstrated that what was actually responsible was the restriction of wheat protein – that is, gluten.

The breakthrough

It was the insight of Dutch paediatrician Willem-Karel Dicke that led to this landmark discovery. It is widely related that he made the observation during the Second World War that coeliac children improved markedly when wheat and rye flours were unavailable and relapsed as soon as supplies were restored to the Netherlands. But he had, in fact, begun to suspect a link to wheat by the mid-1930s, after manipulating the diets of some of his young patients upon hearing anecdotal reports from mothers of the benefit to their children of a bread-free diet.

After years of research, development of his diet, and more formal studies, Dicke became convinced of the value to coeliacs of excluding wheat, and by the early 1950s he had shown that it was its protein – not carbohydrate – that triggered coeliac disease, a fact soon confirmed by other European researchers but that took longer to be accepted in America.

British physician John Paulley realized in 1954 that gluten eroded the architecture of the small intestinal lining, and that this damage could be at least partially reversed by avoiding gluten. In 1956, gastro-enterologist Dr Margot Shiner developed a medical device that could be passed through the mouth, oesophagus and stomach and into the small intestine to allow the removal of samples of its lining. These could then be examined for any characteristic erosion. And so what became the diagnostic technique in the 1960s was developed: biopsy to look for damage, followed by a gluten-free diet, followed by another biopsy to look for improvement, followed by a gluten 'challenge', followed by another biopsy to check for the return of damage. This elaborate process, as unpleasant as it was for the patient, was considered necessary, given there could be other possible causes of intestinal lining inflammation and erosion.

Also in the 1960s, the hereditary nature of coeliac disease was established, as was gluten's link to the coeliac-related skin condition, dermatitis herpetiformis. The Coeliac Society – now Coeliac UK – was founded.

The 1970s and 1980s were characterized by debate and research on the reason for coeliacs' gut sensitivity to gluten. Was it a toxin in the protein? An absent enzyme? Gradually it became recognized that coeliac disease was associated with so-called autoimmune conditions – diseases in which the body's immune system attacks its own tissues – such as type 1 diabetes and thyroid disease. And in the late 1980s and early 1990s, the theory of an immunological basis for coeliac disease was finally accepted: it too was an autoimmune disease, triggered by gluten, and associated with particular gene types.

Blood tests to examine levels of antibodies associated with the disease could now be developed, paving the way towards more convenient ways of making the diagnosis of coeliac disease, and reducing the need for multiple biopsies to just one. Population studies suggested a prevalence much higher than previously believed – closer to one in 100 than one in several thousand – and with that came the appreciation of a huge underdiagnosed population worldwide.

The current picture

Thanks to campaigning from coeliac charities, increased media coverage and the voices of coeliacs themselves, there is undoubtedly a greater awareness of coeliac disease and the gluten-free lifestyle. Specialist gluten-free foods have become widely available, and we have seen remarkable growth in this 'free-from' sector. Food labelling is more precise.

Gastroenterologists now appreciate that coeliac disease manifests itself in a spectrum of symptoms – so much so that it should no longer be looked upon as solely a disease of the gut. Genetic advances – many beyond the scope of this book – continue worldwide. Clinical trials of a number of therapies are under way too, including enzyme pills, vaccines and other treatments. Within ten years, the lives of coeliacs could be transformed. A cure is not out of the question.

How this book will help

We are living in a time of nutritional information overload: never before have we been so bloated with advice on what, how and even when to eat – and why. Increase antioxidants to fight cancer. Reduce tomatoes to ease arthritis. Boost oily fish to relieve eczema. The evidence base for these and other claims like them varies considerably, but the public would be forgiven for thinking that there are any number of diseases that can definitively be treated through dietary manipulation alone. The truth is that there are few.

Coeliac disease is one of them.

In writing *Coeliac Disease: What you need to know* I've taken what we currently know about the disease and tried to distil it into a slim but fact-filled volume. Essentially, it tells you how to find out whether you or your child needs to avoid gluten, how to avoid gluten if one of you does need to, and how to best ensure a healthy gluten-free life.

It covers essentials such as testing and diagnosis – but if you've been diagnosed already and have been given a good grounding in coeliac disease from your dietitian or gastroenterologist, you can jump forward to the chapters on food labelling, diet and nutrition. The psychological and emotional impact of coeliac disease is usually given little coverage – a chapter here addresses that. Some of the recent and exciting developments touched upon above are explained, and their implications outlined. A comprehensive resource section provides links to useful associations and sources of information referred to throughout the book, many of which can offer answers to questions beyond the book's scope.

The book, then, is aimed at several groups of people:

- those who suspect they may have the condition and want to find out more;
- adults or parents of children who have recently been diagnosed with the disease, and need a supportive, practical guide and convenient reference book; and
- long-established coeliac patients who are interested in learning about the more recent developments, and how these may effect them.

Others, I hope, may also find the book useful: those eliminating gluten for other health or lifestyle reasons, loved ones of those with coeliac disease, student or qualified dietitians and doctors, health writers . . .

Note: the abbreviations CD (coeliac disease), GF (gluten free) and GFD (gluten-free diet) are used throughout. (The term 'gluten-free' when used in specific relation to food labelling is not abbreviated.)

Alex Gazzola

1

What coeliac disease is

Coeliac disease (CD) is characterized by inflammation and erosion to the lining of the small intestine – the section of the digestive system that connects the stomach to the large intestine or colon and that helps to digest and absorb food and nutrients.

This damage is caused by consuming gluten – a mix of proteins found in wheat, barley and rye, and therefore in many foods, such as breads, cakes and pastas, that contain them.

CD is not a food allergy, and it is more than just a food intolerance. It is an autoimmune disease. Autoimmune diseases are those in which the body's immune system attacks its own tissues. In CD, these tissues are those of the gut – although other organs may also be affected.

The disease is permanent and presently incurable, but symptoms can be resolved and damage reversed in virtually all cases when gluten is removed from the diet.

(Coeliac is pronounced *see-lee-ack* and is spelled 'celiac' in North America.)

Symptoms

CD can affect many organs and systems in the body, producing any number of a wide range of non-specific symptoms that vary in severity between patients.

Some people have few or no obvious symptoms.

Symptoms in adults

Among the possible symptoms are:

- Digestive – diarrhoea, fatty stools, bloating, wind, abdominal pain, constipation, heartburn, indigestion, nausea, sickness, loss of appetite, weight loss
- Nutritional – deficiency of iron (anaemia), vitamin B12, folic acid and other minerals and vitamins (caused by poor absorption of nutrients as a result of the damaged gut lining)
- Skin and hair – mouth ulcers, dermatitis herpetiformis (an itchy and blistering skin rash), hair loss

- Musculoskeletal – muscle wasting, muscle spasms, joint or muscle pain, osteopenia or osteoporosis (thinning or brittle bones), defective dental enamel
- Nervous system – numbness, tingling in the hands or feet (neuropathy), seizures or epilepsy, unsteadiness or shaking (ataxia)
- Reproductive – delayed puberty, low fertility, recurrent miscarriage, early menopause
- Cardiovascular – irregular heartbeat, palpitations, breathlessness
- Emotional – depression, anxiety, mood swings
- Physical – pallor, tiredness or lethargy, poor growth.

Presentation of symptoms in adults

It used to be the case that the 'typical' adult coeliac patient presented with severe digestive complaints and strong signs of malnutrition, and while doctors still see such patients, these days they are no longer the norm.

Instead, the kinds of people who doctors see have vague, non-specific or non-serious complaints, such as mild tummy upsets, feelings of tiredness, unresolved irritable bowel syndrome (IBS) or a general sense of ill health.

Diarrhoea remains the most common symptom, but it affects only around half of new patients, and it may be sporadic.

Other commonly reported symptoms are tiredness or lethargy (possibly caused by anaemia), weight loss, bloating and abdominal discomfort or pain.

Symptoms can come on so gradually that patients may not recognize that their health is slowly deteriorating. Often, when they do realize it, they may have only a vague sense of when the decline began.

Symptoms in babies and children

Infants and children can present with some of the complaints common to adults with CD, but typical symptoms generally include:

- Digestive – diarrhoea or otherwise abnormal or pale stools, swollen tummy, low appetite or refusal to feed, vomiting, constipation
- Emotional – behavioural problems, tearfulness, irritability
- Physical – tiredness, signs of malnourishment, weak or wasted muscles, stunted growth or inability to gain weight.

Presentation of symptoms in children

Typical childhood CD is characterized by the onset of obvious symptoms at between six months and two years (i.e. soon after the usual introduction of grains), including pale diarrhoea, vomiting, swollen abdomen, muscle wasting, failure to gain weight, and general physical and emotional ill health.

Older children are more likely to have less severe digestive troubles, which may come and go. There may be delayed growth or puberty. There may be defects in tooth enamel, nutritional deficiencies and behavioural problems too.

Teenagers are more likely than other age groups (adults included) to show no symptoms at all, but any of the typical symptoms may present.

Prevalence

Screening studies suggest that around 1 per cent of Western populations has CD.

However, only around 10–15 per cent of those with the disease are diagnosed – meaning that at least 85 per cent of those with CD are unaware and remain undetected. In the UK, this represents around 500,000 people.

Onset and diagnosis

CD can present at any point in life, from six months onwards, well into old age.

Until recently it was believed that the detection of the disease in later life implied a long-standing undiagnosed case of CD, but new research has shown that this is not necessarily true. The disease can be triggered at any age, even after many years of gluten tolerance.

Peak age for diagnoses is among the under-tens and in those aged in their 40s – but increasing numbers are being diagnosed in older age.

The average time for diagnosis in UK patients is a staggering 13 years following the initial reporting of symptoms. Increased awareness among the medical profession and the general public is likely to mean that this figure reduces sharply in years to come.

Susceptibility and risk factors

In recent years, thanks to ever more cutting-edge research, we have come to learn more about who is susceptible to CD and which factors determine whether you may develop it. However, the full picture is not yet clear.

Genetics

Undoubtedly, there is a genetic component to CD. If you have an identical twin with CD, there is at least a 70 per cent chance you will have it or develop it too. If a first-degree relative (parent, sibling, child) has the disease, you are ten times as likely as the general population to have it (a 10 per cent chance). If a second-degree relative (grandparent, aunt, uncle, nephew, niece) has CD, you are twice as likely as the general population to have it (a 2 per cent chance).

In recent years scientists have unlocked more genetic secrets of CD, and we now know that virtually all people who develop the disease have one of two genetic tissue types, called HLA-DQ2 and HLA-DQ8. However, this is also true of around a third of the non-coeliac population, so clearly these genes are required, but not sufficient, for the development of CD.

Other genes that determine immunity, autoimmunity and possibly the functioning of the gastrointestinal system are also likely to be involved, but we don't yet know what these are and how many may be required.

Gluten and diet

Obviously, gluten must be present in the diet for CD to be expressed. Generally, the more gluten consumed, the more severe any symptoms, and possibly the greater the number of types of symptoms experienced.

It is also possible in some cases that the quantity – and, indeed, type – of gluten consumed could be involved in triggering the disease in some individuals. Modern breeds of wheat could be more problematic than ancient and traditional gluten grains, and the form in which they are consumed – typically, as highly processed white flour in bread, pastas, cakes and biscuits – may contribute too.

The age of introduction of gluten into the diet may be a factor as well.

'Leaky gut'

Studies from the USA suggest that patients with CD are more likely to have a so-called leaky gut – that is, an intestinal lining that is more permeable than normal, and that allows incompletely digested food fragments, which are normally excluded from being absorbed, instead to pass through and potentially trigger an immune response in the body.

Trigger events

For most people, there appears to be no clear reason or cause for the onset of symptoms of CD, but in others, it seems connected to an obvious trigger event. It is possible that these events are involved in either triggering the disease itself or in inciting more obvious signs in existing CD that has been previously symptom-free. They include:

- a bout of severe stress
- pregnancy or childbirth
- food poisoning or gastroenteritis – often associated with overseas travel and perhaps with the use of antibiotics
- gastrointestinal surgery – again perhaps with antibiotics.

Disturbance of the gut bacteria population, which helps to maintain gut health, appears to be a common denominator in the obvious triggers. This disturbance could make the gut leakier and increase the likelihood of an immune response.

Other, unknown and subtler trigger events may also be involved. It may be the case that a trigger event is required in all cases – perhaps with the exception of infants who develop CD soon after gluten introduction.

Sex

More women than men are diagnosed with CD, and while it is probable that this goes for undiagnosed cases too (for other autoimmune conditions tend to affect more women than men), it is possible that women are more likely to be diagnosed because they make more visits to their doctors. It may also be related to pregnancy, when immune function is altered.

Underlying autoimmunity

Patients with other autoimmune conditions are more likely to have CD. Around 3 per cent of the population have an autoimmune disease, and around 30 per cent of CD patients have at least one other autoimmune disease.

Type 1 diabetes (insulin-dependent diabetes)

Around 4 per cent of those with type 1 diabetes have CD – that's four times the figure for the normal population.

Autoimmune liver disease

At least 5 per cent of those with one of the several types of autoimmune liver disease will have CD.

Autoimmune thyroid disease

Up to 7 per cent of those with thyroid disease may have CD.

Other autoimmune disease

There appear to be associations with other autoimmune conditions such as Sjögren's syndrome, inflammatory bowel diseases (Crohn's disease and ulcerative colitis), psoriasis, Addison's disease and rheumatoid arthritis.

Genetic syndromes

People with Turner's syndrome, Williams' syndrome or Down's syndrome have an increased risk of CD – as do their first-degree relatives.

The coeliac spectrum

Although previously thought of as a 'black or white' disease – you either had CD or you didn't – this is no longer considered an accurate reflection of the case. We now know that there is a 'spectrum' of manifestations and that it is not clear cut.

Typical coeliac disease

This is the classical version – characterized by diarrhoea, weight loss, malnutrition and, in children, failure to thrive. There is usually quite severe damage to the small intestine.

Atypical coeliac disease

In this form, digestive symptoms may be mild or lacking, and instead there may be symptoms of poor nutrient absorption, such as tiredness, anaemia, irregular heartbeat (suggesting iron deficiency), bone problems (suggesting calcium deficiency) and skin or neurological problems. This is the type more commonly encountered nowadays and these symptoms are often seen.

Silent coeliac disease

This is CD without symptoms, but with underlying damage to the intestinal lining. Silent CD can develop into typical or atypical over time.

Potential coeliac disease

This term is used to describe those patients with a normal gut lining but positive blood (and perhaps other) tests typical of CD.

Latent coeliac disease

A patient, typically a child, who has been previously found (while on a normal diet) to have coeliac-related damage to the intestinal lining that at a later date recovered, and who has since resumed or remained on a normal diet without any relapse, may be said to have latent CD. Regular monitoring is advised.

Dermatitis herpetiformis

Dermatitis herpetiformis (DH) is an intensely itchy skin condition, closely linked to CD, and characterized by blistery, reddened patches, usually on the elbows, knees, buttocks or scalp. It typically affects adults. Like CD, it is caused by gluten, and may be regarded as the skin manifestation of CD – although some consider it a separate condition. Patients may have symptoms of CD too, but most will not. Of this latter group, many are found to have underlying damage to the gut lining or abnormal blood test results for CD when investigated.

Gluten ataxia and gluten neuropathy

These are neurological forms of gluten sensitivity, again closely linked to CD, which have come to light in recent years. Ataxia is loss of co-ordination. A neuropathy causes feelings of tingling and numbness in the hands and feet. Symptoms of CD may be absent.

Other gluten-related conditions

Other gluten-related conditions may be discovered. A link between gluten and schizophrenia, for instance, is being explored.

The biology of coeliac disease

CD mainly affects the top section of the small intestine, a key part of the digestive system. In order to understand what happens in CD, we first need to understand how digestion works.

Digestion

Most food is of no use to the body in the form in which we consume it. In order for it to be of value, it must be broken down into smaller constituents that the body can absorb and reassemble – for instance, to build new cells or to nourish and fuel existing ones. The process of breaking down food is called digestion.

Digestion occurs in the digestive tract (or alimentary canal): the muscular tube that starts at your mouth, takes in the oesophagus (gullet or foodpipe), stomach, small and large intestines, and ends – nine or ten metres later – at your bottom.

The agents that help to break down the food into simpler molecules are called digestive enzymes. Many of the enzymes and chemicals needed for digestion are produced in the salivary glands, the liver, the gall bladder and the pancreas – vital organs, which together with the digestive tract make up the digestive system. Other enzymes are secreted by the cells lining the wall of the small intestine.

At around six or seven coiled metres, the small intestine consists of three connected parts – the duodenum, the jejunum and the ileum – and it is here that most digestion and absorption of food takes place. The upper sections of the small intestine – the duodenum and the jejunum – are the regions typically affected by CD.

What goes wrong in coeliac disease

The inside of the small intestine is not smooth. The innermost layer that lines it is called the mucosa – the gut lining – and this is characterized by a dense array of small finger-like projections called villi. These provide a large surface area available for the efficient absorption of nutrients through the mucosa.

Gluten is quite resistant to breakdown. In people without CD, digested gluten fragments are absorbed and dealt with normally, while undigested gluten fragments pass uneventfully through and out of the body. Any gluten fragments that are absorbed do not appear to pose a problem.

But those with CD aren't so lucky. It seems the lining of the coeliac gut is more 'leaky', allowing gluten fragments through more easily. As people with CD are genetically predisposed to a greater immune sensitivity to gluten, this triggers a response. The reaction is complex, but it is essentially inflammatory and defensive – an attempt by the body to attack the gluten, which it perceives as an invader. The end-result is damage to the villi. Over time the villi can become eroded and flattened, sometimes severely, occasionally totally. This is called villous atrophy.

Untreated, this can cause two key problems. First, the ability to produce digestive enzymes is hampered, meaning undigested foods pass through the system, to get fermented in the large intestine by bacteria, causing diarrhoea, gastric pain and bloating. Second, damaged villi are less efficient at absorbing nutrients, meaning an increased risk of malnutrition and its complications, such as anaemia, infertility and bone disease.

And, as we know, these are the typical signs of undiagnosed CD.

The changing worldwide picture

While the overall prevalence of CD is thought to be around 1 per cent in the West, there are variations among nations – for example, 2 per cent in Finland and 2.5 per cent in Mexico.

Several studies show that the prevalence of CD has increased five-fold, from 0.2 per cent, in the past 35 years, and that it continues to rise, especially among the elderly. The reasons must be environmental, as the genetic status of the population cannot have changed significantly in such a short period.

The problem of CD in the developing nations is serious. It is a common, often undiagnosed and little-known problem in northern India, where wheat is widely consumed (the traditional southern Indian diet is gluten-free), and may be the cause of malnutrition in many children.

Some north African rates can be high, though this problem is a little offset by the availability of other traditional grains, such as corn, millet and sorghum, which probably results in a lower expression of the disease. The Saharawi people of southern Algeria demonstrate a CD prevalence of a staggering 7 per cent and are among those most in need of better medical support.

A case-finding strategy is considered the best way to tackle the so-called CD 'iceberg', by screening all patients with any symptoms possibly indicative of CD – such as anaemia or osteopenia – or with a family history of CD, or who have been diagnosed with IBS (often misdiagnosed instead of CD). One US study showed that the incidence could be increased up to 30 or 40 times with intensive case-finding.

Nevertheless, this is not enough. Several Italian studies have shown that no matter how intensive the case-finding, you can never reach the expected 1 per cent prevalence, and usually attain only 0.5 per cent. This has been proposed by some as a strong argument for mass screening, although this has ethical ramifications.

There are few parts of the world where gluten is not consumed – some south Saharan nations, some parts of the Far East, and New Guinea. Thanks to the general Westernization of the global diet, gluten consumption is likely to continue to rise, and with it the incidence of CD. Undetected cases will cost economies and health services dearly, and this is likely to remain a huge international challenge in the coming decade.

2

Tests and diagnoses

Coeliac disease (CD) can present with many symptoms. If you have digestive and gut problems, a doctor may consider CD, but if these are absent, and you have other general and mixed symptoms – which could easily indicate any number of health issues – it may not initially be suspected. Some doctors retain the outdated idea that CD is a wasting disease, and will not consider it a possibility if patients are, for example, overweight – even though many patients are at diagnosis.

Testing – yes or no?

There are many conditions and situations that may justify testing for CD, and most are now specified in guidelines issued in 2009 by the National Institute for Health and Clinical Excellence (NICE).

Irregular blood test results

Often, routine blood tests for other medical investigations alert doctors to a need for further tests, including those for CD. Irregular blood cells, low iron or calcium levels, or abnormal liver and kidney function markers, for instance, could indicate a problem. In the absence of any CD symptoms, this is how many cases first reveal themselves, but as there are other reasons for these results, it does depend on your medical practitioner pursuing CD as a possibility along with other suspicions.

Common coeliac symptoms

Aside from the well-known digestive symptoms of diarrhoea, nausea, abdominal pain and so on, other symptoms that should be followed up with testing include faltering growth or failure to thrive (in children), sudden or unexplained weight loss, the unexplained presence of anaemia, and ongoing tiredness or fatigue.

Less common coeliac symptoms

Testing should be considered in cases of dental enamel defects, depression or bipolar disorder, epilepsy, certain problems with the bones, unexplained fertility issues and unexplained hair loss.

Irritable bowel syndrome

Irritable bowel syndrome (IBS) is a gut disorder characterized by symptoms such as diarrhoea, constipation, alternating diarrhoea and constipation, bloating, abdominal pain, urgency, incomplete bowel movements and other related complaints.

It is a *functional* gut disorder – a problem with how the intestine works – rather than a *structural* one, in which there would be a physical abnormality detectable by scans, biopsies or examinations.

However, owing to the overlap of symptoms with CD, misdiagnoses of IBS are often made. Recently updated NICE guidelines for the diagnosis of IBS state that tests for CD must now be carried out and CD ruled out before an IBS diagnosis is made with confidence, but if your diagnosis was made some years ago, this may not have been undertaken. It is worth talking to your doctor about this, especially if you have been self-managing your IBS for some years. Research suggests that CD is four times as common in those who have received an IBS diagnosis than in the rest of the population, and hence all IBS patients should have CD tests.

Autoimmune conditions

You should be tested for CD if you have autoimmune thyroid disease or type 1 diabetes.

NICE guidelines state that doctors should 'consider offering' blood tests to those with one or more of several other autoimmune conditions, including Addison's disease, autoimmune liver disease, and Sjögren's syndrome. The incidence of CD among patients with these conditions varies, but averages about 5 per cent. It is usually preferable to test, especially if you have more than one autoimmune condition.

Family history

A first-degree relative – child, sibling, parent – with CD means that you too should be tested.

Chromosomal syndromes

CD is five to ten times more common in those with Williams' syndrome, Turner's syndrome or Down's syndrome, and testing should be considered in these cases.

Before testing

Your doctor should explain several points before you or your child is tested for CD:

- You should *not* stop consuming gluten or feeding it to your child – or reduce intake.
- The blood tests that you or your child undergo cannot diagnose CD on their own.
- Positive blood test results will mean that you or your child will probably need an endoscopy and biopsy (see p. 15).
- Negative blood test results will mean that CD is unlikely, but may not rule out it arising in future.

The necessity of diagnosis

Possibly most important to understand before you undergo testing is why the end-result – a positive or negative diagnosis – is vital.

A confident positive diagnosis is needed to:

- avoid developmental or growth problems that can result with delays in diagnosing or failure to diagnose CD in children;
- ensure that children can subsequently receive care, treatment and monitoring of their development;
- ensure that you receive ongoing care from your doctor and gastro-enterologist (specialist gut doctor);
- avoid the increased risks of longer-term complications of un-diagnosed CD – which include osteoporosis, decreased fertility, undernutrition and a small increased risk of intestinal cancers;
- confirm that a gluten-free diet (GFD) – a tough undertaking – is indeed necessary;
- qualify you for gluten-free (GF) foods on prescription;
- ensure that you receive help and advice from a dietitian on the GF lifestyle; and
- help to alert your first-degree relatives that they have an increased likelihood of CD and should also get tested.

A confident negative diagnosis is needed to:

- help to take your medical advisers a step closer to finding the root of any health problems you're experiencing;
- ensure that there is no reason to restrict your diet unnecessarily; and
- help in part to confirm a diagnosis of IBS – which has its own treatments.

Gluten consumption

Undoubtedly the toughest challenge for many is having to continue to eat gluten – or feed it to their child – prior to testing. Blood testing detects antibodies to gluten, which are produced by the immune system of coeliacs. If you stop eating gluten, the body stops producing the antibodies, and the blood tests won't reflect a true picture. It may be particularly hard to consume bread and pasta knowing that they could be harming you.

The recommendation from NICE and the charity Coeliac UK is to eat 'some gluten in more than one meal every day for at least six weeks before testing'. At least 10 grams of gluten a day is thought to be needed – this can be made up of any combination of, for instance, slices of white bread (2–3 grams of gluten each), or wholewheat bread (4–5 grams each), digestive biscuits or rusks (1 gram each), a small serving of pasta (6 grams), and a Weetabix or Shredded Wheat (2 grams each).

Psychologically, it's important to remind yourself how vital it is for you to do this to achieve the ultimate goal of an accurate result, and potentially a life of health and free of symptoms for you or your child. Try to comfort yourself with the knowledge that it will soon be over and you will have an answer. If you find it difficult, speak to your doctor. In some cases, it may be possible to give your child gluten powder hidden in foods that he or she does not associate with feeling poorly.

Blood tests

Routine blood tests, for instance, to check for anaemia or liver function, can assist a diagnosis and serve to highlight specific health issues, but CD tests are key in the diagnostic procedure. These are very good, but not 100 per cent accurate, which means they cannot usually diagnose the disease alone.

The tissue transglutaminase test

The tissue transglutaminase (tTG or tTGA) test looks for antibodies to an enzyme – tissue transglutaminase – produced when the coeliac-affected gut tries to repair itself.

It is the first-choice test for adults and children and is easy to perform.

When CD is present in adults, it correctly confirms a positive diagnosis in at least 90 per cent of cases. When CD is absent, it correctly confirms a negative diagnosis at least 95 per cent of the time.

The test may be less accurate in children.

The anti-endomysial antibody test

The anti-endomysial (EMA) test looks for antibodies against tissue called endomysium, which joins cells together. It is usually used as an additional test when the results of the tTG test are borderline or uncertain, although it is more expensive and difficult for medical teams to perform.

When CD is present, it correctly confirms a positive diagnosis in 95 per cent of cases. When CD is absent, it correctly confirms a negative diagnosis 99 per cent of the time.

Total immunoglobulin A level

Both the tTG and EMA tests test for classes of antibodies called immunoglobulin A (IgA). Around 2 per cent of coeliac patients have IgA deficiency – natural low levels of this antibody. If the tTG and EMA tests are negative, an IgA deficiency test may be undertaken. If positive, alternative antibodies called immunoglobulin G (IgG) can be used to conduct the tTG and EMA tests instead.

HLA typing

Virtually all people with CD have one of two genetic tissue types – HLA-DQ2 or HLA-DQ8. Testing for these types, then, can also assist a diagnosis – but only in ruling out CD in their absence.

Home blood tests

Personal testing kits are now available. The Biotech Biocard™ Celiac Test, for instance, available from pharmacies, is a kit allowing you to take a small sample of your own blood and test it for coeliac IgA antibodies. The results are said to be as accurate as laboratory results, but of course false positives or false negatives are possible. In practice, there is always the danger that a false negative could offer false reassurance. A doctor is likely to insist on repeating a positive test.

Blood test results

If all blood test results are negative, and there is no other clinical reason to suspect CD, a confident negative diagnosis can be made.

If all the blood test results are negative, but there remains a strong continuing clinical suspicion of CD – typical symptoms, perhaps teamed with strong family history or other autoimmune illnesses – then a referral for a biopsy of the gut lining may be given.

If any of the key tTG or EMA blood test results are positive, you or your child will probably be referred to a gastroenterologist or paediatric gastroenterologist for a biopsy.

However, because it is being increasingly realized that positive antibodies to CD can sometimes be temporary in children, there may be occasional circumstances when it is better to take no action and review the situation in six months or a year.

Endoscopy and biopsy

An endoscopy is an internal medical examination using an apparatus called an endoscope, which is passed into the body.

A biopsy is the removal of a little tissue from the body for examination.

An endoscopy and biopsy of the lining of the small intestine to check for coeliac-related damage is usually considered necessary in diagnosing CD. You or your child will have to attend the hospital outpatients department for the procedure, although young children will need to be admitted and given a general anaesthetic. Food and drink must be avoided for a period beforehand, but check with the endoscopy unit in advance. There may be a need to restrict some medications too. Intravenous sedation is available for those nervous of the procedure. Alternatively, a milder anaesthetic can be sprayed at the back of the throat.

A device is placed into your mouth to keep it open. Air will be passed into your body to expand it and allow the endoscopist to see better. The endoscope, which is a long flexible tube, is passed into the mouth, down the throat into the stomach, and then into the duodenum. The end of the endoscope has a light and a camera, and tiny forceps for obtaining small samples of the lining of the gut. Several samples will be taken from different areas, because the damage caused by CD can be patchy.

Typically the procedure will be over in half an hour. It is entirely painless, though if you have anaesthetic spray it will be slightly uncomfortable. The advantage of the spray over sedation is that you can leave the hospital soon after the procedure. If you are sedated, you will need to wait for several hours, be discharged into the care of a friend or relative, and rest afterwards. You should be back to normal within 24 hours, though you will have a slight sore throat.

The tissue samples are sent to a laboratory for microscopic analysis.

In the case of suspected dermatitis herpetiformis, a small biopsy of unaffected skin is taken.

Is a biopsy necessary?

For some years, the biopsy has been considered the 'gold standard' means of confirming a diagnosis, but improvements in blood testing and in how well CD is recognized among specialists now mean that this view is being increasingly challenged, with some gastroenterologists believing that it may sometimes be better not to put a patient through the procedure.

A study from Derby in 2008 found that tTG test results above a certain level could be 100 per cent accurate in diagnosing CD, and that around 50 per cent of tested cases reached this level – meaning that half of patients could avoid a biopsy and be confidently diagnosed on the strength of the blood test alone. Accordingly, some gastroenterologists have begun to adopt this policy when clinical suspicion is strong and tTG readings are high. Diagnosing without a biopsy is also cheaper and does not add burden to health service resources.

A possible advantage of this from a wider perspective is that it could encourage more people to come forward. Some patients with symptoms may be reluctant to present to their doctor and pursue a diagnosis because of fear of a biopsy.

But there *are* advantages for retaining biopsy as a means of diagnosis. It offers certainty – and some feel nobody should have to go on a GFD if there is any possible doubt.

Some also consider it vital to measure the scale of characteristic gut lining erosion as a 'benchmark'. Should the patient continue to experience symptoms after, say, six months on a GFD, a biopsy may sometimes become essential. Without an earlier one for comparison, it would be impossible to learn how much healing has taken place in the meantime.

The results of a biopsy can also serve as a powerful motivator to stick rigidly to a GFD: without one, a patient may be less likely to appreciate the seriousness of his or her condition and the internal damage that comes with it, and be more tempted to stray occasionally.

This issue is subject to much debate among the coeliac community, and the recommendations are likely to be modified over time, perhaps because of further improvements in blood testing.

Remember that nobody can force you or your child to have an endoscopy and biopsy, and that each case is unique. Discuss options with your medical team.

Video capsule endoscopy

Video capsule endoscopy involves swallowing a pill that has been fitted internally with a tiny camera that takes images as it moves through the patient's intestine. The photographs are transmitted to a receiver worn on a belt by the patient, and these can be downloaded by doctors to look for inflammation or erosion of the gut's lining.

It is not yet approved as a diagnostic technique for CD, and studies on its effectiveness for this purpose have found mixed results, albeit some quite positive. That said, it is becoming increasingly available through the health service.

Diagnosis

Following testing, there are several possible results.

Blood positive and biopsy positive

This combination of results confirms CD.

Blood positive and biopsy negative

This combination of results could indicate absence of CD and false-positive blood test results. A negative HLA typing test can strengthen the negative diagnosis.

This could also be potential CD, however, which can develop into typical or atypical CD over time. It is likely that your doctor will advise you or your child to stick to a normal, gluten-containing diet, and keep the situation under regular review, with perhaps repeat testing in future.

Blood negative and biopsy positive

There are other possible causes of inflammation to the lining – recent gastroenteritis, other gut disorders – and these may need to be excluded. This is especially true of babies and infants, who may have other food intolerances that cause the damage. Generally, though, this result will be viewed as CD, and treated as such.

Blood negative and biopsy negative

CD is currently absent. However, there may be justification to keep monitoring the situation and repeat the blood tests in the future – for instance, in cases of a strong family history or in patients with other autoimmune conditions.

Blood positive and biopsy not performed

If tTG levels are high, and other results suggest CD, this may be enough for some gastroenterologists to diagnose the disease.

It is in infants and babies that there is greater debate regarding performing a biopsy. Some parents may refuse to allow it on their sick children. A cautious positive diagnosis may still be made in these cases, if other criteria are met, such as positive HLA typing and the presence of obvious symptoms (failure to thrive). In this case, a GFD will be recommended, and a diagnosis reinforced if there is health improvement and subsequent negative blood tests.

Testing negative

A negative test may leave you feeling relieved that you don't have CD but frustrated that you haven't found the cause of any symptoms. Rest assured that you are a step closer, having ruled out one of the possibilities. IBS aside, other conditions may need to be considered.

Non-coeliac gluten intolerance

The concept of non-coeliac gluten intolerance remains controversial but is increasingly being accepted by some specialists, as some people in whom CD has been ruled out seem to experience unpleasant symptoms on a regular diet for which relief is obtained on a GFD. It is possible that some may be experiencing nothing more than the health benefits derived from the more nutritionally diverse diet that a GFD may compel patients to follow – rich as it is likely to be in alternative whole grains, fruit, vegetables, nuts, seeds and unprocessed foods – but others may indeed be reacting to gluten in a way not presently understood. This can only be diagnosed through an exclusion diet (see p. 96) under the guidance of a dietitian.

Other food sensitivities

Lactose intolerance is the inability to digest lactose (milk sugar), caused by a deficiency in lactase, a digestive enzyme. Its symptoms are frothy diarrhoea, abdominal 'gurgling', and bloating. Reliable testing (via a breath test) is available, but most other intolerances can only be tested for using an exclusion diet. Children, especially, may be more prone to cow's milk protein intolerance or soya intolerance.

Inflammatory bowel diseases

Inflammatory bowel diseases, such as Crohn's disease or ulcerative colitis, may need to be considered.

Chronic fatigue syndrome or myalgic encephalomyelitis

Chronic fatigue syndrome, or myalgic encephalomyelitis (ME) is an illness characterized by extreme tiredness, muscle fatigue, problems with concentration and depression, and general ill health. Symptoms may include digestive problems similar to those found in IBS and CD.

Invalid testing techniques

There are a number of privately available tests and alternative testing techniques for food sensitivities for which bold claims of their diagnostic abilities are sometimes made by their manufacturers and practitioners. None can diagnose CD, and in fairness the manufacturers may well make this clear. However, reference may be made to 'gluten intolerance', 'gluten allergy' or 'wheat sensitivity', among other food intolerances. The tests include:

- electrodermal or Vega testing (available at some high-street health stores);
- leukocytotoxicity testing (e.g. NuTron, antigen leukocyte cellular antibody test – ALCAT);
- IgG testing (e.g. YorkTest's FoodScan, CNS's Food Detective).

There is no evidence to support the use of the first two, which are regarded as unscientific. There is very little evidence behind the third, and most experts in the field believe it to be of no diagnostic use either.

It is suspected that customers who report improvements after acting on the results and recommendations of such tests are often benefiting from a more nutritious diet. Wheat and dairy are typically identified as problematic foods, and this constrains consumers to cut out all the calorific or junk food in which these two foods happen to be found – pies, pizzas, hot dogs, burgers, doughnuts, cakes, biscuits and so on. These inevitably have to be replaced by more healthy whole grains, vegetables, fruits, dried fruit and nuts. Often, it is the inclusion of these wholesome foods – not the exclusion of theoretically problematic ones – that is the main reason for improved health.

Some complementary practitioners of applied kinesiology, the Nambudripad allergy elimination technique (NAET), homoeopathy and many other techniques may also make claims to be able to diagnose (and possibly treat) food sensitivities. These practices have no place in modern medicine, and have either failed scientific scrutiny or been discredited by researchers. All should be avoided when seeking a diagnosis or treatment of any kind.

3

Food sense: labelling and shopping

The key aspect of successful, long-term management of coeliac disease (CD) is a diet free from gluten. When you are diagnosed you should be referred to a dietitian – or a paediatric dietitian in the case of a child. However, there may be a delay before your first consultation, so you will need to try to get to grips with the basics of the gluten-free diet (GFD) right away.

The gluten-free diet

A GFD is a diet that excludes the following gluten-containing grains:

- wheat
- barley
- rye.

It also excludes:

- all varieties of wheat (e.g. durum, einkorn, emmer, kamut, spelt)
- all forms of wheat (e.g. bran, bulgur, couscous, rusk, semolina, wheat protein, wheat starch, wheatgerm)
- hybrids of the gluten grains, such as triticale (a wheat-rye hybrid)
- some oats and oat products (but see p. 29).

So the GFD must exclude all products containing the grains listed above and all products containing ingredients derived from them – with very few exceptions. It therefore excludes, for example, ordinary breads, pastas, cakes, biscuits, many cereals, and many flour-containing products and pre-prepared meals.

It *includes* all fruit, vegetables, nuts, seeds, non-gluten grains, meats, fish, natural dairy products and eggs, and products and ingredients derived only from these foods.

The wheat problem

Although there are several grains you need to avoid, it is wheat that you'll encounter most regularly. It is widespread in the Western diet, partly because flour-based products such as breads and pastas are staples, and partly because of wheat's additional role as a stabilizer, thickener or 'filler' in processed foods. It may be used to 'dust' products and prevent them clumping together, and can turn up in surprising places. Wheat-based or wheat-containing products may include:

- most flours, breads and baked products – both sweet and savoury
- many cereals
- most pastas, some noodles
- processed meat and fish products – burgers, pies, sausages, pâtés and battered products such as fish fingers
- processed vegetarian products – battered vegetables, pâtés, some tinned soups
- some processed dairy products, such as cheese spreads, thickened milks and creams
- confectionery, including chocolate bars, cereal bars, sweets, chewing gum and liquorice
- miscellaneous products such as stock cubes, gravy granules, condiments and blended seasonings.

Food and drink labelling

Because so many foods may contain gluten, you will need to master the art of reading their labels. Labels on pre-packed products contain vast amounts of information, much of which many people ignore, or misunderstand, or both. As a coeliac, you cannot afford to do either.

Some information is required by law; some is optional. Compulsory information includes the food's name, a list of its ingredients, its weight or volume, its use-by or best-before date, and contact details of the manufacturers – although there are occasional exceptions. Nutritional information is required when health-related claims are made (e.g. 'this is a low-fat product').

Optional information includes serving suggestions, recipes, nutritional information (when no health claims are made), recommended dietary guidelines, and allergy statements or boxes (see p. 23).

Ingredients

The ingredients listing is arguably the most useful section. It presents all ingredients used deliberately in the product's manufacture, in descending order of weight.

The list obviously includes all whole foods. These include names of vegetables, fruits, grains and nuts, for instance. It also includes ingredients derived from whole foods, and whose sources may not be provided or immediately obvious (e.g. 'vinegar' or 'sugar').

Further, the list also may include general collective terms, the details of which may not be supplied or clear either (e.g. 'flavourings' or 'spices') and of course any additives and colourings, possibly as E numbers.

And then there are compound ingredients, which may themselves have their own ingredients, sometimes given in brackets [e.g. 'salami (contains pork, salt, spices, seasonings)'].

Allergens

According to European legislation, certain foods must always be named on the ingredients list – not only when they are present as whole foods, but also when they have been used to manufacture an ingredient or are found in a composite or collective ingredient.

There are 14 such foods or food groups. They are all examples of food allergens. These are foods that trigger food allergies. The best known is peanut, a food allergen that can trigger an allergic reaction in 1–2 per cent of the population.

Although CD is not a food allergy, for clarity and simplicity gluten is often referred to as a food allergen too, and gluten-containing grains are one of the 14 that must be labelled as such.

All the foods and ingredients have been chosen on the basis that they are the most commonly and dangerously problematic ones for people who react to foods. The full list is:

- celery (and celeriac)
- cereal grains containing gluten – barley, kamut, oats, rye, spelt and wheat, or their hybridized strains
- crustaceans (e.g. crab, lobster, prawn)
- eggs
- fish
- lupin
- milk (including milk sugar, or lactose)
- molluscs (e.g. mussel, snail, squid)
- mustard
- nuts (e.g. almonds, cashews, walnuts)
- peanuts
- sesame seeds
- soya beans
- sulphur dioxide and sulphites.

To give an example of a food being used to manufacture an ingredient, let's take 'sugar'. The source of 'sugar' as an ingredient does not need to be specified as 'cane sugar' or 'beet sugar', because neither cane nor beet is on the list of 14 allergens. However, malt vinegar, produced from barley, must say so. This may be represented, for example, as 'malt vinegar (from barley)'. Another example might be 'couscous (wheat)'.

Exemptions

There are some exemptions to this legislation, to allow for derivatives of the 14 allergens that have undergone so much processing or refining that they are no longer considered a threat. As far as the gluten grains are concerned, these exemptions are:

- wheat-based or barley-based glucose syrups, including dextrose
- wheat-based maltodextrins
- cereals used for distillates and spirits in alcoholic beverages.

These are all considered safe for coeliacs. In practice, some manufacturers may declare the source grain – for example, by printing 'wheat dextrose' or 'maltodextrin (from wheat)' or 'distilled vinegar (from barley)' – but this does not mean you need to avoid it.

Note that a single-ingredient product, such as a packet of rye, does not need to carry an ingredients listing, as this is considered obvious.

Allergy information and alert boxes

Although not a legal requirement, many food manufacturers are now adding allergy information boxes to their products. These serve as at-a-glance alerts to the inclusion of any of the 14 allergens – and they emphasize and repeat their presence in the ingredients listing.

The Food Standards Agency (FSA) recommends that if such a box is used, it should mention each of any of the 14 allergens present. For example, if a product declares wheat and peanuts in its ingredients, any box should state 'Contains wheat and peanuts' – and *not* just 'Contains peanuts' (unless the ingredient is an exemption, as above).

However, this recommendation is only 'good practice' and not a legal requirement.

As useful as the allergy box can be, then, do not base a decision about a food's safety solely on it. A good rule of thumb is this: use an allergy box to exclude a food if wheat, rye or barley is mentioned. In their absence, check elsewhere as well.

Ingredient checklist

Ingredients can read more like a list of laboratory chemicals than foods, and you can't be expected to understand all of them. Table 3.1 gives some examples of safe ingredients, and most of the non-safe ones too.

Table 3.1 Safe and non-safe ingredients

Safe ingredients	Not gluten-free
Artificial sweetener	Barley
Aspartame	Barley flour
Carrageenan	Barley malt, malted barley
Caramel	Barley malt extract or flavouring
Cellulose	(unless product complies with Codex
Codex wheat starch (see p. 40)	standard – see pp. 25–7)
Corn flour / malt / starch	Modified wheat starch
Dextrin	Oats, oatbran, oatmeal (unless
Dextrose	confirmed gluten-free – see p. 29)
Distilled vinegar (all)	Rye
Glucose, glucose syrup	Rye flakes
Guar gum	Rye flour
Hydrolysed vegetable protein (HVP)	Wheat
Isomalt	Wheat bran
Maize, maize starch	Wheat flakes
Maltitol	Wheat protein
Maltodextrin	Wheat rusk
Methyl cellulose	Wheat starch (unless it is Codex
Modified starch	wheat starch – see p. 40)
Monosodium glutamate (MSG)	
Rice malt or rusk	
Textured vegetable protein (TVP)	
Wheatgrass	
Xanthan gum	

'May contain . . .' and other warnings

Examples of so-called advisory or 'defensive' labelling include 'may contain traces of wheat' or 'made in a factory which also handles wheat'.

Such labelling may be used by manufacturers for two reasons: to warn the public that wheat (or other allergens, often nuts), although not intentionally added, might have accidentally contaminated a product or one or more of its ingredients somewhere along the harvesting, transporting or manufacturing line; and also to disclaim any liability should a customer suffer a severe reaction.

Manufacturers are advised that advisory labelling should be used only when, following a risk assessment, they believe there is a real risk of cross-contamination.

Coeliac UK says that it can contact manufacturers to talk through the risk, and it does sometimes list such products in its annual handbook, the *Food and Drink Directory* (see p. 30) following discussions with the manufacturers about the production facility and measures to minimize cross-contamination. If you're concerned, contact the charity or the manufacturer for information about suitability. It may well be that the product is all right.

Alcoholic beverages

Alcoholic drinks of greater than 1.2 per cent strength are subject to less strict labelling regulations, and an ingredients list is optional. However, any of the key food allergens must be declared in the name of the product, in a list of ingredients or in an allergy statement or box. In practice, this will usually apply only to brewed drinks – that is, all beers – given that spirits distilled from gluten cereals, such as whisky, are gluten-free (GF) and exempt from such labelling. Most beers will be off-limits to coeliacs, then, but increasing numbers of GF beers are becoming available. For alcoholic drinks weaker than 1.2 per cent, standard labelling regulations apply.

Gluten labelling and Codex standards

The FSA says: 'There is no requirement for gluten itself to be indicated in the ingredient list but if manufacturers choose to use an allergy information/alert box it would be best practice to declare both gluten and the name of the cereal.'

In other words, where you may only see 'wheat' in the ingredients list, you are likely to see something such as 'gluten (from wheat)' or 'contains wheat gluten' in the allergy box, if one is included.

But how is the *absence* of gluten conveyed?

European legislation passed in January 2009 set out strict standards for the use of terms on products that do not contain gluten, and specified that manufacturers comply to these standards by January 2012 (most are expected to be compliant from 2011). They have been brought in for consistency and to help coeliacs manage their risk of exposure to gluten more confidently. Note that these particular rules apply to both pre-packed and non-pre-packed foods alike, and foods from restaurants and other outlets as well.

These vital new standards are known as the Codex standards for gluten, named after an international body, the Codex Alimentarius Commission, created 50 years ago to set up food guidelines.

'Gluten-free'

In practice, it is difficult for manufacturers to achieve an absolute 'zero' level of gluten in their products – and even if they could, zero levels are impossible to confirm by laboratory analysis.

Any products whose ingredients have been processed to remove gluten will usually have residual traces of it – as will some other foods that are naturally free of gluten but that may pick up trace contamination during production processes.

Research suggests that coeliacs can tolerate foods containing up to 20 parts of gluten per million (20 p.p.m. – or 0.002 per cent), with no damage to their mucosal lining or side effects.

Manufacturers can make a 'gluten-free' claim for any product they sell or serve if they can demonstrate that it meets this criterion.

'Very low gluten'

Products containing between 20 and 100 parts of gluten per million (20–100 p.p.m.) can be labelled 'very low gluten' according to the standards. This is more common on products available in northern Europe, and applies to foods whose ingredients have been processed to remove gluten only – not 'normal' foods that happen to be naturally free from gluten, for which a 'very low gluten' claim cannot be made.

Gluten at these levels may cause health problems for some coeliacs, so it is not intended that food in this category be consumed in large amounts, but they are probably safe at least occasionally for many.

'Suitable for coeliacs' and 'suitable for most coeliacs'

These labels may be used to supplement 'gluten-free' or 'very low gluten' claims, respectively – but they cannot be used without them. Alternative phrasing – 'suitable for those on a gluten-free diet' – may occasionally be seen. Coeliac UK's Crossed Grain logo, depicting a line through an ear of wheat, can be used for the same purpose and under the same conditions, if manufacturers purchase rights to use the symbol. Some supermarkets use their own, similar logos.

'No gluten-containing ingredients'

If a food manufacturer or food outlet is unable to confirm 'gluten-free' or 'very low gluten' status for a product – i.e. that it contains 100 p.p.m. of gluten or less – it can instead declare that it does not contain any

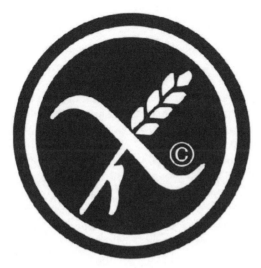

Figure 3.1 The Crossed Grain logo of Coeliac UK. (Used with permission. Registered trade mark to CUK.)

gluten-containing ingredients, provided that it has ensured reasonable steps against unacceptable levels of contamination (steps that it may explain on the label, or make available via leaflets or on its website).

In such cases, claims about suitability for coeliacs or the quantity of gluten present cannot be made, and it is up to individual coeliacs to judge the likelihood of contamination based on available information and any more they can obtain.

Note that because the revised 2009 Codex standard reduced the permissible level of gluten from a previous standard of 200 p.p.m., there may be some foods that were previously able to make a gluten-related claim that from 2012 will no longer be able to. Such foods might, potentially, then carry the 'no gluten-containing ingredients' statement instead. If you have been eating such a product without problem, it is likely you will be able to carry on – but it is worth checking with the manufacturer or Coeliac UK. In some cases the advice may be to swap to an alternative, confirmed 'gluten-free' or 'very low gluten' product.

'May contain gluten'

Manufacturers are advised *not* to use a 'may contain gluten' warning on a product that contains a gluten-containing ingredient (such as barley malt flavouring) but that is able to meet either a 'gluten-free' or 'very low gluten' standard, because this could be misleading.

A question of malt

Malt refers to cereal grains, usually barley, that have been sprouted and then heated and dried. Barley malt or malted barley is not suitable for coeliacs.

The sugar-rich syrup derived from malted grains is called malt extract and its flavouring is malt flavouring. Barley malt extract and barley malt flavouring each contain small amounts of gluten. They are used mainly in breakfast cereals, but also in other foods such as ice creams. Neither is exempt from food labelling and so must always be declared, and 'barley' may appear in an allergy alert box too.

However, in some cereal brands it is used in such small amounts that total gluten levels are below the Codex standard, and therefore considered safe for coeliacs. Coeliac UK devotes a special page to such cereals in their *Food and Drink Directory*. (In this case, the barley may not be declared in the allergy box, as that might confuse consumers.)

Some specialist 'free-from' producers make breakfast cereals such as corn flakes using rice malt or without malt at all.

Some products, such as malted drinks and malt beer, use high levels of malt products and these are unsafe.

Malt vinegar is made from barley malt, which is fermented twice – first to produce a kind of ale, and then to convert it to vinegar. It is used in pickles, condiments and sauces, and like malt extract must be declared. It contains only trace quantities of gluten, and as it is used in such small amounts, it is safe for all but the most sensitive coeliacs.

Malt whisky is safe.

Remember in this case that wheat, rye or barley will have to be mentioned in the ingredients listing, according to food allergen labelling legislation. This is to alert people with a wheat, rye or barley allergy, as opposed to CD.

Additionally, say the FSA, 'Where there is no deliberate gluten-containing ingredient in products labelled as "gluten-free", it is best practice not to use a "may contain gluten" statement.'

'Wheat-free' and 'free from wheat'

This declaration does not necessarily mean free from gluten: the product could contain rye or barley, for example. Sometimes, it is used inappropriately on products containing spelt, which is a form of wheat.

Oats

For the purposes of allergy-labelling legislation, oats are considered gluten grains. However, evidence suggests that the 'gluten' in oats (called avenin) is not toxic to most people with CD (but see p. 42).

It is thought that reactions to oats are more likely to be due to contamination from wheat flour, occurring at some point during harvesting, milling or transportation. Some manufacturers of oats will make a declaration on their products – 'produced in a factory also handling wheat' – telling you that they could be contaminated.

Because single-ingredient products don't need to have an ingredient listing, and because allergy boxes are optional, a packet of oats need not carry any additional information other than its name.

Accordingly, pure and uncontaminated oats manufactured or processed under strict conditions can make a 'gluten-free' claim if they meet Codex standards. Coeliac UK lists such oats and oat-containing cereals in its *Food and Drink Directory*.

Any products using oats as an ingredient and making a 'gluten-free' or 'very low gluten' claim must use oats that meet the Codex standard too.

Food shopping

Shopping for a GFD can be frustrating and time-consuming, but the situation is improving, with increased 'coeliac awareness' of manufacturers, improved labelling protocols and the wider availability of GF foods.

Just been diagnosed? Plan carefully for your first major shop, and go when you have time to devote to it, perhaps during a quiet period when you won't feel stressed. Draw up a list: if you forget to buy a specialist GF product at a major supermarket, you may not be able to find it at your local store. It is important to understand labelling basics before you set off. If you do the bulk of your shopping at the supermarket you can continue to do so: it's unlikely you'll have to change your routine drastically.

The ingredients for everyday GF meals – baked potatoes and beans, rice dishes, 'meat and two veg', homemade vegetable soups – will probably be on your menu, but don't be afraid to try new naturally GF foods.

Been diagnosed a while? Perhaps you're stuck in a rut of eating the same old meals, and haven't evaluated your diet for some time? Again, consider investing more time at your supermarket and other, smaller food stores. You may be surprised at the quantity of alternative and GF food now available.

Food directories

Coeliac UK's annual *Food and Drink Directory* lists around 10,000 safe products and is an invaluable guide. Updated every January, it is divided into sections: prescription products, 'free-from' products, everyday products and supermarket own-brand products. Monthly updates are made available via various means.

It is not exhaustive. Not all companies are willing or able to provide the information required by the charity – even those whose products carry confirmation that they are suitable for coeliacs. Therefore, products not listed in the *Food and Drink Directory* may well be safe. It is important to read labels and, if necessary, it may be worth ringing the manufacturers' helplines for advice. Many manufacturers and smaller supermarkets whose products do not appear in the *Food and Drink Directory* can send you lists of safe foods.

The Coeliac Society of Ireland produce the *Food List*, the Irish equivalent of the *Food and Drink Directory*.

'Free-from' foods

So-called 'free-from' foods are foods manufactured to be free from one or more commonly problematic food allergens that would normally be expected to be present in the food. Usually, this means gluten-free, dairy-free or wheat-free – but egg-free, nut-free and soya-free foods are increasingly popular too.

It is these foods on which you're most likely to find the term 'gluten-free', and many of them feature in Section 1 of the *Food and Drink Directory*. Many supermarkets also have lists of their own-brand 'free-from' foods, which they can send you by post or email.

The 'free-from' sector boomed during the late 'noughties' (the years from 2000 to 2009), with huge year-on-year growth, and many manufacturers now specialize in these niche ranges. Supermarkets, pharmacies and health-food stores stock a range of such products, and in larger branches you'll find 'free-from' sections devoted to foods for restricted diets, including many own-brand foods. Smaller independent stores may also stock them, and will boast more unusual offerings.

It hasn't always been like this. As recently as the early part of the millennium, the selection was pretty grim for coeliacs, with poor-quality breads, which were heavy and grey-tinged and easily fell apart – never mind the odd taste. Now, some of the breads are light, tasty and barely discernible from standard loaves. Then there's the sheer variety: baguettes, ciabattas, rolls, pittas, white, brown, stoneground, multi-grain . . . And it's not just breads: there are abundant GF biscuits, cakes, desserts, flapjacks, noodles, pastas, sandwich wraps, pastries, fish fingers, sausage rolls, pizza bases . . .

Growth is predicted to plateau in the second decade of the century, but innovation and continued demand is likely to keep the market buoyant, as CD diagnoses and interest in the GF lifestyle continue to rise and stronger competition drives further improvement. New technologies – improved methods for 'deglutenizing', for instance – and the bolder use of more exotic GF grains – such as teff and quinoa – hold only promise for the present and future coeliac gourmet.

Such is the interest in the 'free-from' sector that it even has its own awards – the annual Free From Food Awards. Begun in 2008 by Michelle Berriedale-Johnson, editor of food allergy and intolerance portal FoodsMatter.com, winners and nominees have, in recent years, included such innovative products as teff bread flour, cheesebread mix, Victoria sponges, falafel mix, chickpea spaghetti and pastry cases.

Drawbacks

There are downsides to 'free-from' foods, though. First, they can be a little dearer, given that development costs and production methods are more expensive and difficult.

Second, they're not always the healthiest of products. Some can be heavily sweetened and processed and may require a host of additives and preservatives. They're terrific in helping you make the transition to the GFD after diagnosis when everything is confusing and you may be fearful of what you can or can't eat, but it's probably wise not to come to rely on them too much in the long term.

Third, manufacturers are occasionally guilty of making an inappropriate virtue of their 'free-from' status – products proclaiming 'allergy-friendly' should be treated with the same caution as any other food you're evaluating. A wheat-free product may be friendly to someone with a wheat intolerance, but it may also be hostile to a coeliac if it has rye or barley in it. No food is ever wholly 'allergy-friendly'; it depends entirely on the consumer, not the product. Table 3.2 gives a checklist of safe foods, foods that must be checked, and foods that are not gluten-free.

Table 3.2 Food checklist. This table is intended as a guideline to safe and unsafe foods – and foods that usually need to be checked. Never use this list independently of careful reading of the label – which you must always do – because occasional exceptions arise and recipes and production methods change.

Safe	Must be checked	Not gluten-free
Grains, flours, starches Rice, corn and maize, millet, buckwheat, quinoa, sorghum, amaranth, teff Flours and starches made from these grains – such as polenta (cornmeal) – from soya, chickpeas (gram), lentils and chestnut, and from tapioca (cassava), potatoes and other root vegetables (but see *right*) Pure oats	**Grains, flours, starches** Some flours produced from gluten-free grains (see *left*) may be contaminated if milled alongside gluten-containing grains Oats and oat products	**Grains, flours, starches** Wheat (including wheatgerm, bran, bulgur, durum, semolina, couscous, spelt, kamut), rye, barley, triticale, contaminated oats All ordinary flours and flours made from the above grains
Pasta and noodles Pastas and noodles from the above grains and flours, including pure corn pasta and rice or buckwheat noodles Specialist GF pastas	**Pasta and noodles** Some buckwheat noodles or spaghetti may contain wheat	**Pasta and noodles** Italian pastas and wheat noodles
Bakery products Baked goods made from above grains and flours GF bread, biscuits and cakes	**Bakery products** Meringues and macaroons Baking powder Corn tortilla wraps	**Bakery products** All ordinary breads, pizzas, biscuits and cakes
Breakfast cereals GF cereals and muesli mix Pure GF oats	**Breakfast cereals** Corn flakes, rice pops and other malted cereals (see p. 28) Oats and oat mueslis All other cereals not labelled GF and not clearly wheat-based	**Breakfast cereals** All wheat-based cereals (Shredded Wheat, bran flakes)

Safe	Must be checked	Not gluten-free
Meat and fish	**Meat and fish**	**Meat and fish**
All fresh, frozen, smoked and cured pure meats	Meat and fish pâtés and pastes	Meat and fish products in batter or breadcrumbs
All fish and shellfish	Sausages, smoked sausage and salamis	Meat and fish pies and pasties
Pure tinned fish	Burgers	Fishcakes and fish fingers
	Prepared meat and fish dishes and ready meals	Taramasalata
	Tinned meats	
	Sushi	
	Crabsticks and seafood sticks	
	Suet	
Vegetables, fruit and nuts	**Vegetables, fruit and nuts**	**Vegetables, fruit and nuts**
All vegetables and fruit	Prepared salads	Breaded vegetables and tempura
Vegetable oils and fats	Ready-made potato products (e.g. instant mash, waffles, chips)	Vegetarian pâtés
All nuts and seeds and their oils, such as peanut, hazelnut, sesame, sunflower, hemp	Tinned soups and vegetables	
Pure ground almonds	Fruit fillings	
	Roasted nuts and seed or trail mixes	
Dairy products and eggs	**Dairy products and eggs**	**Dairy products and eggs**
Milk, yoghurt, cream, butter, unprocessed cheese	Thickened milks and creams	Scotch eggs
Eggs	Processed, spreadable or cream cheeses	
	Coffee whiteners	
Vegetarian and vegan foods	**Vegetarian and vegan foods**	**Vegetarian and vegan foods**
Plain tofu and bean curd	Veggie burgers	Oat milk
Quorn	Soya-based products	
Vegetarian proteins	Ready-made vegetarian products	
Hummus	Flavoured or marinated tofu	
	Vegetable and nut milks (e.g. soya, hazelnut milk)	
	Soya desserts	
	Vegetable suet	

Safe	Must be checked	Not gluten-free
Drinks	**Drinks**	**Drinks**
Fruit and vegetable juices	Drinking chocolate	Ordinary beers, ales and lagers
Teas, coffees	Herbal teas	Malted drinks
Wine, spirits, cider, GF beers	Cloudy drinks	Barley waters
	Cola drinks	
	Coffee substitutes	
Snacks	**Snacks**	**Snacks**
Rice cakes and crackers	Crisps and related savoury snacks	Pretzels
Natural popcorn	Tortilla chips	
Spreads	**Spreads**	**Spreads**
Honey, jam, marmalade, sugar syrups (treacle, molasses)	Nut butters	—
	Lemon curd	
Yeast spreads		
Sauces and seasonings	**Sauces and seasonings**	**Sauces and seasonings**
Vinegar (including malt)	Stock and stock cubes, bouillon	Chinese soy sauce
Herbs, pure spices, garlic, salt and pepper	Packet sauces, jarred sauces	
	Relishes, mustard products, marinades	
	Mayonnaise and salad cream	
	Blended seasonings	
	Curry powder, mix and sauce	
	Japanese soy sauce	
	Worcestershire sauce	
Sweets and desserts	**Sweets and desserts**	**Sweets and desserts**
Jellies	Chocolate products	Semolina puddings
Meringue	Confectionary	Ice cream cones and wafers
Most dark chocolate	Ice creams	
Sweeteners	Ready-made desserts	
Sugar	Liquorice	
	Custard powders	
	Blancmanges	
	Mincemeat	

Other foods

Plenty of foods not specifically aimed at coeliacs will of course be suitable. Some may not make a gluten-specific declaration because the manufacturers can't afford or do not wish to pay for rigorous testing or the Crossed Grain symbol.

Thousands of such foods are listed in section 2 of the *Food and Drink Directory* – divided between branded foods and supermarket own-brands.

Product recalls and food alerts

Mistakes can occur in food manufacturing. Products can be mislabelled, or can get contaminated with food allergens and find their way on to the shelf before the error is detected. When noticed, though, the food industry leaps into action, and there are several ways in which messages will be conveyed to consumers.

Manufacturers may take out advertising in national newspapers, explaining the nature of the problem, the batch number or product code of affected foods, and advice on what to do if you have bought the product. Their websites will also carry the warning, and many issue email newsletters to customers – so if you come to rely on certain companies' products, register with them or subscribe to their bulletins. (These tend to apply more often to nut contaminations, owing to the sometimes life-threatening nature of nut allergies.)

Read any conspicuous signs in supermarkets, recalling products, which may be located at checkouts or customer service counters or where the products in question are stocked.

Coeliac UK's website carries all product recalls issued that are of concern to coeliacs. The FSA issues food alerts, including allergen alerts. Click to <www.food.gov.uk/enforcement/alerts>, where you can read and register to receive them.

Non-pre-packed food

The grey area remains non-pre-packed food sold loose at bakeries, salad bars, butchers and deli counters, for instance. Contamination may be a possibility here, by virtue of close storage, handling, or a 'wandering' spoon or knife. Cheese products may be sliced on or alongside machinery also used to slice, say, breaded ham, transferring contaminants between the two. If you can't be confidently reassured by staff, it is best to avoid such foods.

The new gluten standards *do* apply to non-pre-packed foods, so any that do meet these standards will be permitted to carry the 'gluten-free' message on the counter. However, many will be unable to meet the stricter standards that will be in place by 2012, and might instead make statements such as 'no gluten-containing ingredients'. Again, you must check with staff whether you can be reassured enough that the product is safe.

International foods

Although wheat is the dominant grain and source of starchy carbohydrate in Western society and cuisine, it isn't in many overseas food cultures, in which it may be used much less frequently. Markets, stores and delicatessens devoted to international cuisines can offer an eye-opening array of foods for you to explore, albeit perhaps when you are feeling more adventurous and settled into GF life. Check out Japanese soba (buckwheat) noodles, Mexican mesquite flour, Korean sweet potato vermicelli, Chinese bean curd noodles, Vietnamese tapioca sticks . . .

Shopping online

The major supermarkets now act as internet retailers too and their sites allow you either to tick a 'free-from' box in order to filter out non-'free-from' foods and/or specify GF, or to enter 'gluten' in a search string, which should reveal available GF foods. Ingredients for items are shown and many carry allergy-related information too. Even Amazon. co.uk has branched into selling GF products.

The advantages of shopping this way are clear: it's time-saving, you can browse at leisure at all hours and you can buy long-lasting and heavy food products in bulk and have them delivered.

Weighed against this must be delivery costs, and perhaps having to plan ahead what you want to eat over coming weeks. It's also not quite the same as browsing and examining a product close-up – unless you've bought the product before, it's not always easy to know what you're getting.

Online 'free-from' retailers, specializing in products for all those on restricted diets, are thriving. Check deliveries carefully when they arrive, though, as mistakes can happen.

Online 'cottage' industries

There has been remarkable growth in the number of small, often home-based or family-run businesses, operating mostly online, whose 'shop front' is essentially their website's home page.

Many are owned and staffed by coeliacs, who understand the needs of those on the GFD all too well. Quality is usually high. Products are often hand-made, using mostly natural and sometimes locally sourced ingredients, low in additives. Some offer personal and 'bespoke' services – for instance, cakes for special celebrations, incorporating other dietary needs too (e.g. soya-free, nut-free).

Many are so small-scale, though, that they may not be able to afford tests needed to demonstrate they meet the Codex standards for gluten labelling, even if the ingredients they use do meet them, and they maintain a working environment free from gluten. Word of mouth and online chat forums are a great way to source recommendations.

4

Food sense: eating and dining

In Chapter 3 we learned about the gluten-free diet (GFD), food label-ling and food ingredients, and the variety of specialist 'free-from' food available. In a sense, that was the 'food sense' *theory*.

Now comes the *practice* – actually putting that knowledge of safe foods to work on your eating and dining lifestyle and habits. And there's one person who can help you in this regard more than anyone else.

Your dietitian

When you are diagnosed with coeliac disease (CD) you should be referred to a registered dietitian – a trained and qualified professional who can help to translate the science of nutrition into personalized practical dietary advice and guidance. Dietitians are understanding and supportive, and many specialize in restricted diets or food sensitivities. A child with CD will see a paediatric dietitian.

It is important you see your dietitian regularly and build up a strong relationship because evidence shows that those regularly in touch with their dietitians stick more rigidly and healthily to the GFD in the long term and have more satisfactory health outcomes.

Your first appointment

In the days leading up to your first appointment, keep a one-week food diary of everything you or your child eats and drinks, and when. Your dietitian will want to know about your diet in order to help best plan replacement foods and meals that are nutritionally adequate, and a diary will give a more accurate reflection as your memory can be unreliable.

Take a list of questions with you. Take notepaper and don't be embarrassed to write down answers. Your dietitian will give you lots of information, but you will not remember it all, although he or she will supply you with leaflets.

During the appointment your dietitian will go through a number of key issues with you:

- what gluten and CD are and how both affect the body;
- gluten-containing foods, safe foods, food labelling, food shopping and the implications of the GFD;
- gluten-free (GF) products available on prescription (see below), the companies that produce them, and perhaps some samples or vouchers;
- aspects of health – weight, symptoms, any improvements or problems since diagnosis, exercise, smoking, alcohol intake, etc;
- any dietary restrictions – vegetarian, co-existing food allergies; and
- cooking and eating out (see pp. 42–51).

One of your dietitian's key aims will be to impress upon you the value of the GFD and how quickly you will start to feel better once you exclude gluten. Yes, there may be ups and downs, but the overall trend over the months to come will be of health improvement, possibly starting within days, as your gut mucosa begins its road to recovery and becomes more efficient at absorbing nutrients. Digestive symptoms should ease, as should any tiredness and depression, for instance.

A common concern at this early stage is that you will need a radical overhaul of your diet. Again, a dietitian can explain that this will not need to be the case, that lots of foods are naturally free from gluten, and that the availability of palatable replacement products will mean that your staple meals need not alter drastically – GF pasta can replace wheat pasta; GF breads can replace ordinary loaves.

And, of course, many of these will be available on prescription.

Prescription food

Anyone diagnosed with CD is entitled to a limited number of certain GF products on prescription, and a dietitian can offer advice in this regard. Your dietitian may stress that it is important to take advantage of this entitlement, as research shows that compliance with the GFD is helped by access to prescription foods, and he or she may point out that, quite often, prescription products are healthier and lower in fat or sugar than their supermarket 'free-from' counterparts.

In Ireland, some prescription items are available to those with medical cards, although others can claim tax reliefs.

Available products

Products that are available on prescription include breads, bread flour, cake mixes, baking aids, crackers, pizza bases, pasta and plain biscuits. There are various brands to choose from, with different qualities for different tastes, and the list changes occasionally, with new products added and others removed. The *Food and Drink Directory* itemizes available products, and Coeliac UK's website has a downloadable list and can alert you to updates. The list of products is approved by an independent body, the Advisory Committee on Borderline Substances (ACBS), and it is from this list that your doctor can usually prescribe.

In trying to court new and potentially lifelong consumers, many of the key suppliers of 'free-from' and prescribable foods will send you 'welcome packs', samples or vouchers of products to try.

There are guidelines for the quantities that can be prescribed: in the case of your child this is based on his or her age, and in your case it is based on age, sex and level of activity and, if you're a woman, on whether or not you're pregnant or breastfeeding. The recommendations are given as monthly 'units', with children being entitled to anywhere between ten and 18 units, and adults between 12 and 20 units. One unit is equivalent to 250g pasta, 400g bread, two pizza bases or 200g biscuits or crackers, for example.

You can usually, within reason, use your allocation as you wish, although a doctor will not allow you an unhealthy balance of many units on items such as biscuits. Take your dietitian's advice when discussing your initial prescription: he or she may recommend, for instance, products with a higher calcium content if you are calcium-deficient, or foods that can be frozen, or advise against heavy ordering of products with short shelf-lives, all depending on your personal circumstances. Your dietitian can also make a case for you if he or she feels your unit allowance should be increased for any reason.

There may, however, be some restrictions, depending on the area of the country in which you live. The budgets for prescriptions are managed by the local Primary Care Trust (PCT) and cutbacks may influence what your GP may prescribe. Any local health initiatives may reduce the availability of biscuits and cake mixes too. Contact Coeliac UK if you think your prescription has been restricted unfairly.

Codex wheat starch

Ordinary wheat starch is not GF as it has enough residual gluten to cause problem for coeliacs, but there is a special type of wheat starch that is permitted for use in foods labelled 'gluten free' or 'very low gluten', and it is almost exclusively encountered in some prescription foods.

The starch is commonly called Codex wheat starch – or just 'Codex' among coeliacs – a specially rinsed starch whose trace gluten level complies with Codex standards, making it suitable for use in products such as breads and flour mixes that comply to these standards. Most, but not all, coeliacs can tolerate the trace levels in these foods.

Manufacturers like to use it as it can offer better taste and baking qualities and a lighter texture. It will always be specified on the label.

Some coeliacs are concerned by the methods employed to 'deglutenize' the wheat starch, but the only chemical involved in the (repeated) rinsing process is water.

Getting started

Your doctor will write and sign your prescription, based on the products you have selected within your entitlements, and you can take this to your community pharmacist who will order your food and dispense it to you.

The early months will be in some ways experimental. You can tweak your prescription accordingly, again with the help of your dietitian. Repeat prescriptions are possible, but it's better to wait until you've worked out a selection of foods and a routine that works for you.

There are pharmacy-led local prescription schemes in some parts of the UK.

Cost

Prescriptions are free for children and for some adults, depending for instance on age, income or geographical location. Pregnant women and those with some long-term health conditions do not pay either.

If you do pay, it may be cost-effective to opt for a pre-payment certificate (PPC), available for either three months or 12 months, which offers unlimited prescriptions. This helps if you pay for other prescriptions as well as your GF entitlements or if you order a variety of product types on prescription, as usually one charge is applied to each 'line'.

Controversies and issues

Most, but not all, coeliacs obtain food on prescription, and it is a personal decision whether you choose to do so. Some people don't like the medical connotations of 'illness' that a prescription implies, while others choose mostly to abandon a diet of processed food products and cook their own meals exclusively from scratch with ingredients naturally free from gluten.

The use of Codex wheat starch in prescribed foods is criticized by some coeliacs who feel that wheat should be excluded completely from foods labelled 'gluten-free'. Others feel that they react to Codex, and indeed some more sensitive coeliacs do appear to have to avoid it. These may include children, who may find the levels less tolerable.

Those who have to follow a wheat-free or dairy-free diet in addition to a GFD may be unfairly limited in their choice. Some feel that biscuits, and even some of the more calorific, higher-fat breads now available on prescription, should not be prescribable from a health perspective. These issues are vigorously debated and discussed within the coeliac community, and the situation is changeable.

If you do settle into a repeat prescription for GF foods, you may encounter such problems as a sudden change to your prescription in the event of cutbacks, or the lack of availability of some products, perhaps depending on your pharmacist. It is worth calling Coeliac UK if you feel unfairly treated, as they may be able to take up your case.

Oats in the diet

Uncontaminated GF oats are considered safe for the majority of coeliacs, including children. But it is currently impossible to predict who the few who may react may be, and so the recommendation is that following a diagnosis, you should refrain from consuming oats for around 12 months, until symptoms have improved and blood tests normalized. Speak to your dietitian before introducing them.

Cooking

There is certainly more to coeliac-friendly cookery than merely boiling some rice for your stir-fried vegetables or popping a baked potato into the oven to go with your beans. But before you don your apron and get cooking more adventurously, there are considerations to take care of first.

The GF kitchen

If you live alone (or perhaps exclusively with other coeliacs) then you will be able to benefit from 'deglutenizing' your kitchen. Previous baking with ordinary flour might mean there's suspicious white powder lurking in corners, and perhaps breadcrumbs too, so a thorough washing of all kitchen equipment and surfaces is advised.

Toasters can be tough to clean so you will need to replace yours. As for food, give any gluten-containing products to non-coeliacs. Think carefully about where breadcrumbs may be hiding: honeys, marmalades, margarines and other spreads may have crumbs in them if you've 'double dipped' your knife after first applying it to the bread or toast.

The non-GF kitchen

Cross-contamination is a major issue if you are either cooking for non-coeliac family members or sharing with others in a non-GF household.

You will have to be more scrupulous with cleaning, and communicate this importance to the rest of the household. If you can, foster a 'tidying up as you go' approach, rather than allowing unwashed pots and pans, half-eaten bits of food and assorted ingredients to build up, only for gluten to get picked up on fingers and spread further. It will be much easier to keep on top of matters if the kitchen is tidy.

You won't need separate kitchen utensils or other equipment, for the most part. You may need an allocated toaster (although you can use toaster bags), a slicing or chopping board, a bread maker and a bread bin. Reserved cake and biscuit tins are essential. It's wise to have different drainers for different pastas, as drainers can be tricky to clean properly. You'll also need a no-gluten item of any equipment that isn't washed but, say, just 'wiped' clean – such as a wok. Dishes, bowls and cutlery, provided they are washed properly, will be safe.

That said, some coeliacs do like to have total separation of GF and non-GF, virtually splitting the kitchen into two. Certain products that may be easily mistaken for one another, such as plain biscuits, or that may easily cross-contaminate, such as flours, should be stored separately. Use of prominent labelling or a 'colour-coding' system – perhaps red for non-GF and green for GF – can help here.

It can also help with food: labels on leftovers or for freezer items can avoid confusion. Separate margarines and other spreads are recommended. The alternative is a rule where nobody 'double dips' a knife – you included. It may help to go for 'squeezable' options – such as plastic bottles of honey – which can't be contaminated.

Care must be taken when preparing gluten-containing and coeliac-friendly meals at the same time: avoid using the same spoon to stir two different pans of boiling pastas, for example. It's wise to maintain clear separation during cooking. If you have the time, it's better to prepare the coeliac meal first. Regular hand-washing, taking care under nails and jewellery, is paramount throughout.

A lot of the time, once you've taken basic common-sense precautions, you may find that it's best to devise the rules as you go along, learning from trial and error. It may be frustrating at first, but you will get there.

Should the household give up gluten?

There are advantages and disadvantages to this.

The advantages include easier, quicker and cheaper shopping and less cooking (with no risk of cross-contamination).

The disadvantages are that the GFD is 'imposed' on one or more non-coeliac family members, who may resent it. In the case of children, this could cause problems. Many feel that coeliac children should not be shielded from the realities of a gluten-containing world in this way and that they should learn how to deal with it at home.

A compromise could be best: go GF where you can, make mealtimes mostly GF, encourage non-coeliac family members to take an interest in GF cooking and take care with cross-contamination issues. Most sweet bakery products are equally good in GF forms.

It is ordinary bread and pasta that non-coeliacs are unlikely to feel they can sacrifice, and these should be accommodated with the usual precautions. Self-contained gluten snacks – such as cereal snack bars – are fine if stored separately and clearly marked for consumption only by non-coeliacs.

Meals

Avoid if you can thinking of and focusing on the limitations of the GFD – all the foods that you can't cook with and eat. Try to concentrate on what you *can* eat instead – and look upon it as an opportunity to broaden your culinary palate. Truthfully, having to replace gluten staples with GF varieties and getting to experiment with grains naturally free from gluten can open your eyes to a new world of food. Approach it with a sense of adventure, think creatively, and don't be afraid to make mistakes. You will learn from them. And get better.

Favourite recipes

We all have favourite meals, and there are few recipes that cannot be adapted for coeliacs. For instance, although rice or chickpea spaghetti bolognese or bread and butter pudding made with GF bread may not taste *exactly* the same as the regular recipes, and your tastebuds will take a few weeks to adapt, try not to think of these adapted meals as 'not as good as' they were – just 'different from'. Rest assured that GF versions for most ingredients now exist, so you can find replacements for anything you need.

Great grains

It is important on a GFD to replace the grains you can't eat – wheat, rye, barley – with the cereals or cereal-like foods you can. You're already likely to be eating rice and corn, and will probably be familiar with polenta or cornmeal, but there are others, and each is nutritious and tasty in different ways.

- Amaranth – a tiny grain, a key crop to the Aztecs. It has a nutty taste, is easily digested and high in proteins, calcium, magnesium and iron, making it ideal for vegetarians and vegans. Cooks in about 15 minutes and should not be overcooked as it quickly turns gooey.
- Buckwheat – despite the name, it is not a wheat, and is definitely free from gluten. Popular in Japan, pure buckwheat noodles (soba) make a good alternative to rice noodles and a good substitute for spaghetti. The seeds come in raw form (green) and roasted (reddish-brown). It is commonly used in parts of Russia and China, has a sweet taste, and can be used in casseroles or as a substitute for couscous.
- Millet – slightly bland cereal of tiny spherical grains, a staple in Africa. It should be cracked by sautéing before cooking, so that it can absorb flavours. Millet flakes can be used as an alternative to oat porridge. It is highly digestible.
- Quinoa – an ancient South American crop, quinoa is a high-protein, complete food, which is nutty, and cooks in 15 minutes, turning into tiny translucent 'beads'. Use instead of rice or couscous.
- Teff – native to eastern Africa, and popular in Ethiopia, teff is a tiny, mild and nutty grain, which can be used in soups and stews, as a substitute for bulgur wheat or as an alternative to porridge. It is a nutritious source of iron, calcium, magnesium and zinc.

New recipes

This isn't a cookbook, and it's beyond its scope to include recipes. Over time you will want to try new meals. You can find ideas from a number of sources:

- existing cookbooks, from which recipes can be adapted;
- specialist coeliac, GF or 'allergy-friendly' cookbooks, of which there are an increasing number;
- Coeliac UK's website and magazine, *Crossed Grain*;

- FoodsMatter.com – a resource devoted to people with food sensitivities;
- coeliac (or celiac) and GF blogs – there are many of these, run by 'foodie' coeliacs; and
- coeliac chat forums, support groups, etc.

Baking

You don't have to bake. It can be tough to get right, requiring patience and practice. Gluten imparts elasticity and doughiness and 'bind' to regular bread – making it light, airy and cohesive. Without it baked products can turn out dense and friable.

GF breads are so much tastier than they used to be. Ordinary bakers are branching out into baking for coeliacs, and quality is likely to improve further with increased competition and developments in molecular science. The standard of some smaller speciality producers is exceptional.

If you do want to bake, consider ready-made bread or flour mixes,

Flours naturally free from gluten

There are many flours that are naturally free from gluten, each with unique characteristics, and you will come to have your own favourites. Here are a dozen, with some suggested uses, although most are more versatile.

- Arrowroot – good for thickening both savoury and sweet dishes
- Buckwheat – for pancakes and crepes, and noodles
- Chickpea or gram – for savoury Indian and Asian dishes and flatbreads
- Chestnut – for sweet baking (cakes, biscuits)
- Cornflour – a thickener, for battering, as meat coating; corn pasta
- Mesquite – for sweet recipes or flatbreads
- Potato – a savoury thickener (for soups, sauces); for pancakes and waffles
- Rice – in all baking and as a thickener; to make rice noodles
- Sorghum – for Indian breads and sweet bakery; coating for fried foods
- Soy – for egg-free baking; pancake mixes
- Tapioca – for sweet and chewy breads and desserts; for thickening sauces
- Teff – for savoury breads and sweet cakes.

many of which are available on prescription, and just require you to add some staple ingredients.

The bolder will want to be more creative and experimental, perhaps invest in a bread maker, and look at experimenting with various flours. A key ingredient in GF baking is a vegetarian starch called xanthan gum, used to replace the characteristic elasticity of gluten. GF baking powder is widely available.

Good results from baking cakes and biscuits is easier – and fun . . .

Eating out

You can't always eat food prepared in your newly safe GF kitchen. There will come a time when you will want or need to consume food prepared by people you don't know. Dining out is one of life's great pleasures, and you shouldn't deny it to yourself. For many, picking up a quick bite for lunch is a normal part of their working day, and business dinners and family social events are regular events for lots of us.

That said, mistakes are more likely when you're away from home, so it's not something you can treat lightly or be overconfident about. It is vital to understand what you can and cannot eat – it's no good expecting others to if you don't.

Restaurants

Clearly this presents a challenge and a risk, so pre-planning is vital. That said, more chefs and establishments are aware of CD and understand that it is not a fad. You may even find some dishes labelled 'gluten-free' – remember that labelling rules will also apply to these foods from 2012.

Before you dine out

- Ask for recommendations. Fellow, long-standing coeliacs will know of good places, and a local coeliac group will be able to make suggestions.
- Check for a website. Most restaurants and restaurant chains have a website, with their menus online, and may have reserved areas for those on special diets.
- Phone ahead. Speak with the head waiter or chef. Try in mid-afternoon during a quiet period. Ask whether those on a GFD can be catered for, and what may be available.
- Give examples. Explain which kinds of meals are naturally free from gluten or easily adapted to a GFD, such as rice-based meals and meat, fish and vegetable dishes.

- Explain cross-contamination. Give staff an example of how this may occur: a wandering stirring spoon between the rice and pasta, for example, or the re-use of oil that has already been used to fry some breaded products.
- Convey the severity of your condition. Sadly, not everyone takes food sensitivities seriously, possibly because many fad dieters and celebrities casually claim to be 'allergic' to various foods. Don't just say 'I can't eat gluten,' use powerful words: 'I have coeliac disease' or 'Consuming even a trace of gluten will make me extremely ill.'
- Get family, friends and colleagues 'on side' before you go out. Let them know about your dietary needs and that you will need to talk about them, so you don't feel embarrassed when the time comes, and they can support you as needed.
- If you're not comfortable with the arrangements and don't feel re-assured that you can be safely catered for, then change your plans.

Once you arrive

- Ask to meet the person you spoke with. Go through your conversa-tion again, confirming what you've agreed, reminding the other person of how serious CD is, about cross-contamination issues and of the need to check labels on products such as stock cubes, bouillon or sauces that the chef may be using.
- When you arrive at a restaurant at which you haven't pre-booked, inform a member of staff immediately about your requirements. Ask if they can check whether there are safe foods available. Don't be shy of articulating the precise consequences of errors. Ensure that your conversation is witnessed by members of your party. If you are not confident that the seriousness of your condition is appreciated, don't eat there.
- Read menus carefully. Never let hunger or impatience get the better of judgement. Ask waiting staff to clarify ambiguities and specify safe meals – possibly recommended by the chefs.
- Don't be shy of questioning staff precisely. Is the chef 100 per cent certain of all the ingredients he uses in his recipe? Might a food be cooked in oil previously used to cook an unsafe food? Are separate chopping boards and knives used to prepare different foods? What are the ingredients of the dressings? Have the 'safe' desserts been stored alongside others? Listen carefully to replies.
- Don't become complacent. Go through the usual checks in restau-rants in which you've previously dined and have come to 'know'. Suppliers, ingredients, chefs, recipes and menus all change. Check every time.

- When your food arrives, use your eyes and nose. Does it look all right? Never pick croutons out of salad, for instance – send it back. Re-confirm with waiting staff that your meal is safe: in busy restaurants, with many clients to attend to, instructions can be forgotten and mistakes made.
- Be polite throughout. Make a point at the end of the meal of thanking staff for catering for you. It will encourage them to become more aware of those with specific dietary needs. Further, spread the word and report excellent establishments to others.
- Remember: it's OK if you don't want to go through this rigmarole. Understandably, there will be times when you may not want to wear your 'coeliac hat'. A bit depressing, perhaps, but in this instance plain food is safest – like meat and vegetables, or a baked potato and cheese. Soups, stews and other dishes where ingredients are easily disguised or hidden are best avoided.

Other eateries and takeaways

Obviously, there are other places where you'll eat: places you may not want or be able to ring up beforehand.

The 'chippie'

Of course you can avoid pies and battered fish, but it's cross-contamination in the oil used for frying chips that's the key issue here. Some chip shops have special evenings for coeliacs.

Fast-food chains

Some of the popular fast-food chains' products are listed in the *Food and Drink Directory*, and these chains will gladly give you a list of GF food served.

Pubs

Some pubs have a GF menu.

The 'Italian'

Italian restaurants are often coeliac-unfriendly, with pizza and pasta galore. Some pizzerias will add toppings to your own GF pizza base – but you must stress that it needs to be baked in a clean oven. Some chains have 'allergy charts' on their websites.

The Chinese takeaway

Wheat noodles and soy sauce are an obvious source of gluten, but there's also the problem of the tradition of not washing a wok, causing possible cross-contamination.

The Indian takeaway

Traditional Indian cooking – especially from the south – is largely, but not totally, GF. But watch out for traditional breads like naans. Chickpea flour is the usual thickening agent, though, which is naturally free from gluten. Ask about cross-contamination of deep-fried foods.

The sushi bar

A lot of sushi is naturally free from gluten, but you need to check. Check the soy sauce too.

The sandwich or salad bar

Some sandwich bars have GF sandwiches. In salads, any grain should be checked, but gluten may be hiding in dressings too. Those bars that allow you to make up your own salads and choose your own dressings are the safest.

Coffee and tea shops

These increasingly stock GF sweet treats.

'Eating out' labelling

The European regulations on the labelling of foods for coeliacs that are coming into full force in 2012 (see p. 25) also apply to foods bought in restaurants, takeaways, delis, cafés and other eateries. In other words, food products with under 20 p.p.m. of gluten can be labelled 'gluten-free' and those under 100 p.p.m. 'very low gluten'. Supplementary claims – such as 'suitable for coeliacs' – may also be made in these cases. The FSA says, 'These claims can be made, for example, on menus, blackboards, or in discussions between the customer and the serving staff.' Outlets will have to put forward their foods for analytical testing before claims can be made, and they will subsequently have to be able to demonstrate that controls remain in place to maintain such low levels of gluten.

There is a concern that smaller outlets will not be able to afford the testing required on their foods and meals to satisfy the legislation, limiting options for coeliacs. The FSA says, 'If they do not contain any gluten-containing ingredients, and producers have made every reasonable effort to minimize cross-contamination, factual statements can be made about the presence/absence of gluten-containing cereal ingredients – for example "no gluten-containing ingredients" – provided they do not indicate suitability for those with a gluten intolerance or mention levels of gluten. These statements will help coeliacs make informed choices and prevent further restriction of their diet.'

Dining at friends'

Being invited to dinner and having to inform your hosts of your condition can feel awkward, but you must impress upon them its seriousness. You may have to explain CD from 'scratch' – what gluten is, where it is found, food labelling, cross-contamination issues, places in which wheat 'lurks' (such as sauces and stock cubes) and so on. It may feel more trouble than it's worth, but good friends will be accommodating and do their utmost to help. Go easy on them: it can be a lot to take in, and some may make mistakes.

Don't be shy of enquiring what your hosts are planning to prepare: 'May I ask what you're thinking of serving? I'm afraid my severe intolerance to gluten restricts what I can eat.'

You could ease your discomfort by offering to help with preparations and cooking, or by offering to bring your own safe ingredients or prepared dishes that can be microwaved.

5

Food sense: diet and nutrition

It is natural to feel anxious about the impact your diagnosis has had on your nutritional status, and about the ongoing effects of your new dietary limitations on your well-being. But it is perfectly possible to eat well on a gluten-free diet (GFD) – and you may find you eat more healthily than before.

Eating a healthy diet

So much is written nowadays about eating healthily that you can easily become overwhelmed with the unnecessarily detailed and sometimes contradictory advice given. It's easy to form the impression that nutrition is complicated. It isn't. In reality, sticking to a few basic principles should ensure that you maintain good dietary habits.

Possibly the most important principle of the GFD is variety: try to eat as diverse a diet as possible. You may not want to spend time fretting over which food offers which nutrient, but you can obtain a wide range by mixing it up as much as possible. Avoid coming to rely on any one 'safe' food that provides only a limited range of nutrients; overconsumption can also increase your risk of becoming intolerant to a food.

How you eat is vital too. Take your time – when you're selecting food, preparing it and most importantly eating it. Eat when you're calm and relaxed and can focus on your meal, not when rushed or distracted, as mistakes are more likely then. Remain quietly vigilant and on guard – always. Take care not to become complacent about eating habits – continue to check labelling and to monitor your diet.

Also, don't skip meals, especially breakfast – you'll experience uncomfortable fluctuations in energy and blood sugar levels, and you'll be more vulnerable to casual snacking and grabbing possibly unsafe convenience foods on the go. Plan ahead, and always have good safe foods to hand in case you should be caught short and feel peckish during the day.

Essential foods

Several food groups are key to your daily diet.

Complex carbohydrates

These include all grains, such as rice, quinoa and millet, and the foods based on them, such as gluten-free (GF) pastas, breads and cereal products. Potatoes also fall into this category. Roughly eight to ten daily servings for teens and adults and approximately four to seven for children are required to ensure an adequate intake of slow energy-releasing carbohydrates and of fibre. A slice of GF bread, an egg-sized potato, three tablespoons of GF muesli and two heaped tablespoons of cooked rice approximate to a serving each.

Protein foods

Two to three servings of meat, fish, eggs, beans, nuts or seeds are advised. A portion is equivalent to 100g of meat or fish, two eggs, three tablespoons of beans or a handful of nuts and seeds.

Fruit and vegetables

Fruit and vegetables are essential sources of carbohydrates, fibre, vitamins, minerals and antioxidant chemicals, and you should aim to consume at least five portions daily, preferably more, and in a variety of colours. A handful of berries, an apple, a banana, three tablespoons of peas or lentils, and two heaped tablespoons of salad are roughly equivalent to one portion.

Dairy foods

Two or three servings of either milk, yoghurt or cheese are recommended by dietitians. A matchbox-sized chunk of hard cheese, a small pot of yoghurt or a glass of milk each provide a serving. Avoid too much cream or butter, as these are high in fat.

Healthy fats

Some fats are needed in the diet, and these may come from some of the foods mentioned above. Unsaturated fats – found in fish (especially oily fish), nuts, seeds, avocados and vegetable oils such as olive oils – are the best.

Water

Two litres daily is the often-quoted figure to which we should supposedly all aspire, but the quantity depends on so many factors – the size of the person, the amount of activity undertaken, the temperature and environment – that it's misleading to generalize.

A good barometer of healthy and adequate hydration is the colour of your urine: too dark signifies that you may lack fluids, so aim to drink enough to keep your pee straw-coloured. Water itself is the best hydrator, but fruit juices, squashes, sodas and milk all contain mostly water and count towards your quota, as do, within reason, teas, coffees and colas. The dehydrating effects of the caffeine in these drinks are hugely exaggerated by many complementary nutritionists but research shows they are negligible. Alcoholic drinks, which dehydrate heavily, certainly do not count.

The eatwell plate

The eatwell plate is an FSA pie chart representing the proportions of food groups that you should consume in a healthy, balanced diet. It can be viewed at: <www.eatwell.gov.uk/healthydiet/eatwellplate>.

The eatwell plate principles can be applied to the GF diet, and the approximate percentage shares to aim for are:

- Fruit and vegetables – 33 per cent (i.e. one-third)
- Natural and rendered sources of carbohydrates (potatoes, rice, other GF grains, GF breads and GF pastas) – 33 per cent (one-third)
- Dairy products – 15 per cent (one-seventh)
- Protein-rich foods (i.e. meats, fish, eggs and pulses) – 12 per cent (one-eighth)
- High-fat and high-sugar foods – 7 per cent (one-fifteenth).

Non-essential foods

In moderation, other foods are permitted in the context of a healthy GFD, but take care not to overindulge.

Convenience and snack foods

It's wise to limit your intake of junk foods, desserts, sweet products and processed snack foods, partly because they are high in saturated fats.

Trans fats are a particular class of fats manufactured during hydrogenation – a process that converts liquid vegetable oils into solid fats and margarines – and they are often used to prolong shelf life. They are unhealthier than saturated fats, offer no contribution to nutrition, and are linked to high cholesterol and cardiovascular disease. Typically, trans fats are found in pastries, cakes, biscuits, convenience meat products such as pies and sausage rolls, and some takeaway foods. Be wary of 'free-from' foods listing hydrogenated or partially hydrogenated vegetable oil or fats on the label, as these may contain trans fats. Many manufacturers have a 'no trans fats' policy.

You should also take care with the salt content of nibbles such as crisps (which aren't always free from gluten). Salt can dull the taste buds and contribute to high blood pressure.

Sugary treats

Cakes, biscuits, pastries, chocolate bars, sweets – most of us love occasional treats, and they may be important for your psychological health, especially if you're feeling down about having to exclude gluten. Eat sugar sparingly, though – no more than 10 per cent of your daily calories should come from sugar, which is roughly equivalent to 50g or 12 level teaspoons. Read labels carefully for added sugars.

Caffeine

Moderate caffeine consumption is safe for most adults, but avoid drinking more than four cups of coffee daily in order to stay within recommended guidelines, and remember that black and green teas, cola, cocoa and chocolate products all contain caffeine.

Alcohol

Moderate alcohol consumption – up to two or three units a day – is generally considered fine for most adults, and although you may be advised to abstain for a while after your diagnosis while your gut heals on the GFD, there's no reason why you won't ultimately be able to enjoy spirits, wine and GF beers. The health risks of excessive alcohol consumption aside, as a coeliac you do need to take extra care as drinking can reduce your vigilance – it's easy to thoughtlessly pop a pretzel from the bar into your mouth when you've had a few more than you should.

'Free-from' foods

These have their place, and can be useful, but some products may contain high levels of refined carbohydrates, fats and additives – notably the 'treat' foods. The best products are likely to be the staples found on prescription, some of which are fortified with nutrients.

Coeliac nutrition

Getting you off a gluten-containing diet is the priority when you are diagnosed, but establishing yourself on a nutritionally complete diet comes a close second – joint with the need to resolve any nutritional deficiencies stemming from poor food absorption due to your damaged gut lining that may have been caused by a delay in your diagnosis. These may have been picked up during the diagnostic process, but your dietitian may order further blood tests to get a current picture.

Some minerals and vitamins of particular concern are discussed here.

Calcium

This is a vital mineral for healthy teeth and bones and, as a result of poor absorption, you will possibly be deficient in it, and have a need for higher levels in your diet. Your dietitian may also recommend supplements. Long-term low calcium intake can put you at risk of osteoporosis (brittle bones) in later life (see p. 66).

Coeliac children do not have an increased need above the ordinary recommended levels.

Foods rich in calcium are:

- All dairy foods
- Fortified GF flours and breads
- Fortified soya products and tofu
- Fortified vegetable milks
- Leafy green vegetables
- Beans and pulses
- Seeds and nuts
- Bony fish.

Iron

This is a vital mineral for healthy blood and, again because of poor absorption, you may well be iron-deficient and have anaemia. This is of particular concern in teenage girls and young women. Your dietitian is likely to recommend supplements to normalize your iron levels, but will also suggest iron-rich foods to incorporate into your diet.

Foods rich in iron include:

- Red meat (the richest source)
- Oily fish
- Egg (especially the yolk)
- Fortified GF breads and cereals
- Amaranth and quinoa
- Dried fruits, such as figs and prunes
- Dark green vegetables
- Lentils and chickpeas
- Soya and tofu
- Nuts and seeds.

The absorption of iron can be reduced by tea and coffee, so avoid these with or soon after meals. Absorption can be helped by vitamin C, so it's good to drink juice with an iron-rich meal.

Magnesium

Deficiency in this mineral is common, not only in newly diagnosed coeliacs but in the wider population too. Magnesium is essential for the formation and maintenance of bones and tooth enamel, and deficiency can increase the risk of brittle bones.

Foods rich in magnesium include:

- Fish, meat and dairy products
- Amaranth, buckwheat and quinoa
- Green vegetables (e.g. spinach, broccoli)
- Nuts and seeds
- Beans and pulses.

Zinc

This is a 'wonder' mineral in that it has many functions in the body, and many newly diagnosed coeliacs may have compromised levels. It is essential for the digestion of food, for growth and body tissue repair, for immunity and defence, and for sexual health.

Foods in which zinc is found are:

- Red meat and poultry
- Eggs and dairy products
- Shellfish (e.g. oysters, lobster, crab)
- Nuts, especially Brazil nuts
- Soya and other beans
- Wild rice.

B vitamins

The many B vitamins have abundant roles in the body, and there has been concern that coeliac diets are naturally lower in them, because substitute products such as GF cereals do not contain as high levels as regular cereals because they are less likely to be fortified with B vitamins.

Folate (folic acid)

Deficiency of this particular B vitamin, common in coeliac disease (CD), may contribute to anaemia, because it is involved in the production of blood cells. Foods in which it can be found include:

- All green vegetables
- Corn
- Pulses, chickpeas and beans
- Oranges
- Wild rice and millet.

Vitamin B12

Needed for growth, development and the healthy functioning of the nervous system, vitamin B12 is required in conjunction with folate to produce blood cells, so a deficiency, which is an occasional problem in CD, can also lead to anaemia. Vitamin B12 is found in:

- Meats and fish
- Eggs and dairy products.

It is not found in naturally vegan foods, so if you don't eat animal products, alternative sources are:

- Fortified soya foods and vegetable milks
- Fortified yeast extracts
- Fortified margarines.

Vitamin D

Deficiency in vitamin D is another common problem in coeliacs. The vitamin is needed, with calcium, to optimize bone health. It is made in the body by the action of sunlight on the skin, and so a little light exposure daily is important. Good food sources include:

- Oily fish
- Eggs
- Fortified vegan foods (milks, 'cheeses' and margarines).

Vitamin boosts – supplements and injections

Your dietitian will probably recommend that you take some nutritional supplements, at least for a short period. Avoid supplementing without specialist advice, never assume you can compensate for omitted foods with vitamin pills, and don't use supplements as substitutes for skipped meals. Always verify that supplements are free from gluten – your dietitian can advise. Never take additional supplements without letting your dietitian know.

In more serious cases of deficiency, injections of vitamins – for instance, of vitamins B12, D or K – may be recommended.

Weight management

'Classical' CD patients are often underweight, but these days 'atypical' forms of CD are more commonly encountered among those newly diagnosed, and it is being realized that many patients are of average weight – or even overweight – at diagnosis.

Once established on a healthy GFD, many coeliacs start to put on weight. This should be generally interpreted as a healthy sign: the gut lining is healing, and becoming more efficient at absorbing nutrition and therefore calories. With health improvement comes appetite improvement, further driving caloric uptake.

But if you are overweight, or if you become overweight, it is a cause for concern, as this can have implications on long-term health and increase your risk of type 2 diabetes and cardiovascular disease.

There is a wide perception that the GFD is automatically healthy, largely as a result of celebrities in the media, who speak about having lost weight after giving up gluten. In the everyday world, this is not necessarily the case.

There are obviously steps you can take to control your weight, or lose weight if you need to, and your dietitian can advise. He or she will probably recommend at least light to moderate exercise: activity is hugely important.

Low glycaemic index foods

The glycaemic index (GI) of a food is a measurement of how it affects your blood sugar levels.

Some foods, those with high GI scores, are digested quickly by the body and so increase blood sugar levels rapidly. In an attempt to 'normalize' these levels, your body releases large quantities of the hormone insulin into the blood. But this can cause a sudden 'dip' in blood sugar, leaving you hungry and lacking in energy. And the result is you eat more.

Instead, many dietitians recommend that you should concentrate on foods with moderate to low GI scores. These tend to be those that your body has to work harder to break down, and that therefore release energy into the blood slowly. These foods are more sustaining and satisfying over a longer period, making it less likely you'll be tempted to eat between meals or make your subsequent meal a larger one than needed, helping with weight control.

High GI foods

These should be consumed in moderation, and include white rice, baked potatoes, sugars, sweets, refined GF cereals, GF treats, white bread and chips or crisps.

Moderate GI foods

These include whole grains (e.g. quinoa, brown rice), GF muesli or oats, GF pasta, new potatoes, sweetcorn and a few fruits.

Low GI foods

Examples include brown GF breads, all pulses and lentils, nuts, seeds, dairy produce, most vegetables and many fruits.

Notable from these lists is the high GI value of some of the default GF staples that people typically turn to when diagnosed: white rice and baked potatoes. This is why it's important to incorporate non-gluten grains into your diet.

Fibre

There is some evidence that coeliacs eat less fibre than non-coeliacs, and that some GF replacement food is lower in fibre than the regular food. Fibre adds bulk and 'fill' to the diet, helping with weight control. Some tips:

- Choose whole grain GF cereals with, for instance, amaranth and millet.
- Go for brown versions of GF pasta, breads and pizza bases if you can.
- Whole grains such as brown rice, buckwheat and quinoa are important sources of fibre.
- Flours made from gram or chickpea and buckwheat, for example, are more fibre-rich than ordinary GF white flours.

If boosting your fibre intake, remember to keep up your fluid intake.

Sweet treats

Some research indicates that adult female coeliacs have a slightly higher average energy consumption than non-coeliac women, and that this difference is due to sugars in the diet. It is possible that women may be more likely to 'treat' themselves or to overcompensate for the restrictions of a GF diet with more sweet foods. 'Free-from' sweet foods may be more calorific.

Obviously, you need to moderate your intake of sweet and high-fat and calorific treats, which should make up no more than 7 per cent of your daily intake. This means a small piece of GF cake or a few GF biscuits. It's better to restrict them to after a meal, so they don't cause a steep rise in your blood sugar levels. Of course, for occasions, you can enjoy (a little) more.

Weight loss

Weight loss is possible if, as a newly diagnosed coeliac, you find the GFD difficult, unpalatable or depressing. Some people feel wary or suspicious of consuming prescription foods made from Codex wheat starch, or even safe foods, so closely do they relate their diet to their ill health. Understandably, many are frightened of eating out.

Your dietitian will address this with you if he or she notices a problem, but speak to him or her if these feelings are familiar. Your dietitian can also help to reassure you of the safety of GF products, increase your confidence and understanding of food labelling so you can choose food confidently, and introduce you to alternative foods, with advice on recipes. A GF cookbook can also inspire you.

Here are some ideas to boost calorie intake in a healthy way via energy-dense, naturally wholesome foods:

- Add seeds and crushed nuts to yoghurts and salads.
- Fortify smoothies with protein powders (e.g. hemp, flax).
- Add rich cheeses, olives and avocado to salads.
- Enrich soups with cream or grated high-fat cheese.
- Stir chopped dried fruits into GF oat porridge.
- Avoid diet or low-calorie products such as diet colas.

Probiotics

Billions of bacteria live on the lining of your gut. Weighing in total around a kilogram, these bugs keep your immune and digestive systems working well, and help you to digest and absorb vital nutrients, as well as neutralizing any toxins. These so-called 'good' bacteria – or probiotics – also ward off 'bad' bacteria – the pathogens that can cause infection and poisoning.

Research suggests that those on the GFD have slightly poorer populations of gut bacteria, and that coeliacs are more likely to have an overgrowth of non-beneficial bacteria in the gut, which could be responsible for ongoing symptoms.

Because modern diets contain few naturally occurring probiotics, there is now a range of food products fortified with them. These include yoghurt products and milk drinks.

The most common probiotics on the market are from the *Bifidobacter* and *Lactobacillus* families, which some experts have suggested offer us better general benefits than other bacterial families and which also seem able to survive the acidic environment of the stomach and the various digestive processes, to reach the large bowel, where they are needed. Studies suggest that they can help to reduce bloating, speed up a sluggish digestive system and support the immune system, but it is becoming increasingly clear that different probiotics have different qualities and can help with different conditions.

There has been some modest research on the possible benefits of probiotics in CD. A Finnish study published in 2008 found that the probiotic *Bifidobacterium lactis* could counteract the toxic elements of wheat gluten and possibly inhibit them from triggering damage to the gut lining. Researchers suggested that probiotics could have value in accelerating gut healing after beginning a GFD, and perhaps even serve as an ongoing protective mechanism against coeliacs' almost inevitable low-level gluten intake.

A Spanish study from 2010 found that *Bifidobacter* probiotics may offer strong anti-inflammatory benefits to the coeliac gut.

Even though the case for probiotics is far from proven, there is unlikely to be any harm in boosting your diet with them. Supplements are available, but dietary sources include:

- Live yoghurts
- Fortified yoghurt drinks and fermented milk drinks
- Sauerkraut
- Miso (check that it is rice or soya miso, not barley miso)
- Tempeh.

Prebiotics

Whereas *pro*biotics are bacteria which promote health, *pre*biotics are indigestible carbohydrates, naturally found in some foods, which feed those friendly bacteria already in your bowel and encourage their proliferation.

A fruit- and vegetable-heavy diet will be richer in prebiotics than a processed- or meat-heavy diet. The known prebiotics are fructo-oligosaccharides (FOS), inulin and galacto-oligosaccharides (GOS). They are found generously in chicory and Jerusalem artichokes, and to a lesser degree in garlic, onion, leek, asparagus, GF oats, beans and bananas.

Resistant starch is thought to have prebiotic properties too. Resistant starch is a type of starch that is not fully digested in the small intestine and that reaches the large intestine where it becomes available to probiotics. It occurs in cooked cold potatoes, green bananas, cold brown rice, beans, pulses, oats and yams.

6

Health issues

In addition to your nutrition, you may also be concerned about other health implications of your diagnosis, of which there may be several.

Other autoimmune diseases

Having an autoimmune disease such as coeliac disease (CD) increases the likelihood of having others. Some are quite rare, but a few of the more common ones are considered below. Symptoms should be referred to your doctor.

Dermatitis herpetiformis

As dermatitis herpetiformis (DH) is a part of the coeliac spectrum, a gluten-free diet (GFD) is the key treatment, but the rash will not clear up quickly with diet alone. A drug called dapsone can help to get the itchiness of the rash under rapid control, but you may need to take it for up to two years. The side effect of anaemia is fairly common, so this will need to be monitored. Dose reduction can be considered after six months once treatment and the GFD are established.

Type 1 diabetes

This is an autoimmune disease in which the insulin-producing pancreas is damaged. Insulin promotes the body's uptake of sugar from the blood. In its absence, the sugar remains in the blood and does not get used for energy. Symptoms of increased thirst, frequent urination and tiredness result.

Type 1 diabetes is typically diagnosed in childhood, and almost always before a CD diagnosis when they co-occur. Around 4–5 per cent of people with type 1 diabetes have CD.

Blood glucose (sugar) control is the cornerstone of treatment, and this will include a diet high in low or moderate GI foods (see p. 59).

One concern to those with diabetes is the level of sugar in some 'free-from' products, but it's a myth that people with type 1 diabetes have to give up sugar or sugary foods, although they should be only occasional treats in the context of a healthy diet.

Many people with type 1 diabetes find their glucose levels rising when they move to a GFD, but this is likely to be because their healing gut is absorbing more food. This may mean that you need to adjust insulin replacement quantities.

Epilepsy

This is a neurological condition characterized by recurrent seizures triggered by episodes of increased electrical activity in the brain disrupting normal 'communication' between cells.

CD is slightly more common in people with epilepsy than in the general population, and a possible link between autoimmunity and epilepsy has been explored since the 1980s.

There are anecdotal reports of people with epilepsy experiencing fewer, or even no, seizures once established on a GFD.

Thyroid disease

The thyroid is a gland in the neck, which produces hormones that regulate metabolism, thermoregulation, nervous system functions, cardiovascular functioning and more. There is a strong link between autoimmune thyroid conditions and CD, and it is worth being aware of possible symptoms and discussing these with your health-care providers should they arise. Stress or pregnancy may be a trigger in some cases.

Graves' disease

This can cause overactivity of the thyroid gland – also known as hyperthyroidism. It is most common among women in their 30s and 40s. Its symptoms are varied and include:

- weight loss
- irritability, feeling emotional
- dislike of heat and warmth
- increased sweating
- swollen thyroid, presenting as a swelling in the neck called a goitre
- bulging eyes or swelling around eyes
- shaking, tremors and rapid heartbeat
- thinning hair.

Hashimoto's disease

This causes chronic thyroid inflammation and underactivity of the thyroid – also known as hypothyroidism. There may be only mild symptoms, if any at all. Others have more notable symptoms, including:

- tiredness
- weight gain
- dislike of cold temperatures
- muscular and joint pain
- slower heart rate
- goitre
- brittle hair and scaly skin
- constipation.

Rheumatoid arthritis

A weak association between rheumatoid arthritis and CD exists. Symptoms are:

- painful / swollen joints
- stiffness in the morning
- weak grip
- tiredness and feverishness.

Sjögren's syndrome

In this relatively common autoimmune condition, the moisture-producing glands in the eyes and mouth are attacked. Other organs may also be affected. Symptoms include:

- dry mouth and sore tongue
- dry and itchy eyes
- vaginal dryness
- digestive problems
- joint and muscular pain.

Crohn's disease and ulcerative colitis

These are serious inflammatory bowel disorders, whose symptoms are similar to those of CD and can be mistaken for a relapse in the condition. Severe diarrhoea or gastrointestinal malaise must always be referred to a gastroenterologist.

Multiple sclerosis

This is caused by autoimmune damage to the nerves of the central nervous system. It produces symptoms such as:

- tingling and numbness
- blurring of vision
- balance and movement problems
- muscular weakness
- tiredness.

Other autoimmune diseases

There are almost one hundred autoimmune conditions in total, some extremely rare, with a battery of diverse symptoms, from jaundice and enlarged liver (autoimmune hepatitis) to hazy vision (auto-immune uveitis). There are some symptoms that are common to several of them:

- joint or muscular pain or weakness
- feeling hot/sensitivity to cold or heat
- low fertility and sex drive
- digestive problems
- co-ordination problems and dizziness
- palpitations or an irregular heartbeat
- tingling in the hands and feet
- memory and concentration problems
- depression or mood swings
- dryness of the skin, mouth or hair.

Osteoporosis

One of the most serious and important long-term health considerations in those diagnosed with CD is osteoporosis – a condition in which the bone mass and density is reduced and bones are more liable to fracture. A huge risk factor is poor absorption of calcium, required for healthy bones, in years of undiagnosed CD.

It is diagnosed via a dual-energy X-ray absorptiometry (DEXA) scan at your local hospital, and this should be advised in those at risk, in order to measure bone mineral density. People at risk include post-menopausal women, men aged over 55 years, the underweight, anyone who has experienced previous fractures and those with a family history of the condition. You are more susceptible if you smoke, drink excessively, take little exercise or have a low-calcium diet.

There are a number of recommendations by which you can reduce your risk:

- Stick rigidly to a healthy, calcium-rich, GFD.
- Take regular exercise – including weight-bearing exercise.
- Keep to a healthy body weight.
- Keep to within safe alcohol consumption limits.
- Quit smoking.
- Take supplements of calcium or vitamin D, or both – but only if recommended by your doctor or dietitian.

Hyposplenism

This is a reduction in the functioning of the spleen – a small organ on the left side of the abdomen that helps protect against bacterial infections. Hyposplenism is more common in those with CD.

Hyposplenism is usually picked up via blood tests, and your health practitioner may advise you to be immunized against certain infections to which you may be more vulnerable because of it. The injections may include the flu jab, the pneumococcal vaccine, and the *Haemophilus influenzae* type B (Hib) vaccine.

Medical treatment

It's likely at some point that you will need to receive medical care unrelated to your CD.

If you or your child have to be admitted to hospital for any reason, be aware that your medical team may have very little awareness of CD. Coeliac UK advises you to plan ahead, as some hospitals can find it difficult to cater for those on a GFD. Speak to the charge nurse of your ward or the hospital's dietitian to find out what the hospital can do and whether you need to bring in your own foods. If you don't call ahead, it may take the hospital some time to obtain gluten-free (GF) supplies. Be vigilant about any food served to you or your child, and always check it is safe. Anaesthesia has no gluten, and most medicine should be safe too, but always let medics know, just in case. Take some back-up food supplies, and your *Food and Drink Directory*, which may be useful to staff.

By all means let your dentist know you are a coeliac, but there is unlikely to be any product your dentist uses in your mouth that contains gluten.

However, owing to the association between dental enamel defects and CD, especially in children, it is worth letting your child's dentist know about a coeliac diagnosis.

7

Emotional well-being

When there is so much to take on board as a newly diagnosed coeliac – the food-labelling rules, the new food and diet regime, the various physical implications and so on – the psychological impact of your diagnosis may take a back seat. As so much of your time is occupied with the practical implications of your condition, it's easy to neglect your emotional health. So what problems can manifest themselves – and what are the possible solutions?

Coping with diagnosis

Some people welcome their diagnosis. Perhaps after having suffered for years, with doctors unable to get to the root of the problem easily, it can be a relief to be told that the problem isn't all in their heads and is real, and that a gluten-free diet (GFD) should put them on the road to recovery.

But others don't cope so well. 'Why me?' you may wonder. 'Is it something I did wrong?' Remind yourself that nobody is to blame for coeliac disease (CD): you, or your child, just got unlucky. It was genetics combined with a trigger over which nobody had control.

In an ideal world, as a new coeliac you would react 100 per cent positively, take the diagnosis on the chin, arm yourself effortlessly with a wealth of knowledge on the condition, and experience no emotional hiccups in making the transition to a gluten-free (GF) lifestyle.

But this is real life, and most people, through no fault of their own, find the road to acceptance a bumpy one, much like a bereavement.

Shock, anger, disbelief

You may feel fury that your body has let you down, perhaps that you're still young, that it shouldn't be 'failing' you already. You may find the diagnosis difficult to believe, and the implications too huge to contemplate: 'It cannot be true!' Perhaps you feel anger at the situation in which you find yourself, anger at how much you're going to miss out socially and food-wise, anger at the glutenous society, filled as it is with newly banned foods such as pizzas and cakes, which have suddenly become unavailable to you. You may take your frustration out on loved ones.

Letting your feelings show can be beneficial in the short term. It is normal, and it will usually pass quickly, and those close to you will, it is to be hoped, understand.

Denial and indifference

'I don't have to worry about reading labels or watching what I eat – my partner or mother will make sure I eat the right things.'

'I know I've got to cut down on gluten – but I can still have a few biscuits with my tea in the afternoon.'

'I've managed fine up till now. I can put up with the diarrhoea, take some Imodium, and will just carry on as before. It can't be very serious.'

Do you recognize any of the above attitudes?

Passing the buck for your care on to others, not taking the diagnosis seriously, adopting a reckless attitude towards your well-being – these are all possible initial responses that need to be tackled, especially if they linger.

Self-pity

A brief period spent feeling sorry for yourself can do you good: if you're overwhelmed with your diagnosis and its implications, having a short 'shut down' for a few days could be just what you need, and is perfectly normal. Allow yourself time off work. When you emerge from the gloom, as you begin to accept your situation, you will probably find yourself ready to face the task head on.

Ongoing problems

Some people take CD in their stride. Others experience occasional or chronic psychological difficulties, and it is vital to be aware of these.

Depression

This is a symptom of undiagnosed CD, but one study found that diagnosed coeliacs on a GFD were more likely than the general population to be depressed. A short period of mild depressive withdrawal can act protectively. But when this stretches on indefinitely, the situation becomes serious.

Older people, a group in which diagnosis rates are rising sharply, may be particularly susceptible to the 'coeliac blues'. You may be feeling doubly fragile at a time when your body might already be showing other signs of 'wear and tear'. This vulnerability can be much more debilitating than the practical implications of suddenly having to avoid wheat. Feeling 'set in your ways' and unable to make adjustments may also bring you down.

Symptoms of depression include:

- indifference, including to pleasurable activities
- reduced appetite or reduced interest in food
- lethargy and tiredness
- disordered sleep patterns
- poor concentration and motivation
- feelings of inadequacy or hopelessness
- loss of self-confidence.

Complacency

This is a sign that denial could be creeping back. Ask yourself these questions:

- Have you taken to being cavalier with checking food labels?
- Are you beginning to take risks with products carrying 'may contain' warnings?
- Have you started to catch yourself wondering, 'I've been healthy for ages – how much can it hurt, just this once?'
- Do you increasingly avoid telling people about your condition when you should?
- Have you skipped appointments with your doctor or dietitian?

A 'glutening' episode can act as the wake-up call in this situation, but it is preferable to identify any slide towards complacency, and nip it in the bud.

Lingering denial

'I've been gluten-free for three months, so I deserve that piece of cake.'

'I wasn't very ill. My body will have recovered now and I'm young and healthy so it doesn't matter if I stray every now and then.'

The problem with ongoing denial about the realities of CD is that it can, clearly, lead to cheating on the diet and exposing your gut to gluten. Naturally, it's tempting. You may desperately miss bread. You may get offered a piece of birthday cake in the office and want to enjoy it with everyone else. It's very, very hard.

Embarrassment

Sadly, many coeliacs feel ashamed of their condition, and embarrassed at feeling as if they're 'making a fuss' at social events. People are not always understanding or sympathetic: because the GFD is undertaken by some people as a means through which to lose weight or 'detox', you may be treated sceptically as a dieter or faddy eater.

Coeliacs can react to this in one of two ways: either they avoid social situations and isolate themselves, or they expose themselves to risks by not speaking up.

Anxiety and stress

Even if you were relieved at your diagnosis, that relief may be short-lived: the stress of not knowing what was wrong and perhaps trying to convince your doctor that something was amiss may have been lifted, but now it has been replaced with the anxiety of an uncertain future. How are you going to cope? *Can* you cope?

Some underlying anxiety is OK: you need to be alert to possible danger and ready to respond. For instance, it is vital that you maintain a low, constant level of vigilance to avoid gluten, so don't look upon stress as all bad.

That said, chronic stress can be debilitating: it is often felt in the gut – the last place you want disturbance as a coeliac – and is a sign of a problem that needs to be addressed.

Symptoms of anxiety include:

- a dry mouth
- cold or hot sweats
- changes in eating habits
- inability to work or concentrate
- sleep disturbance
- sexual disinterest or dysfunction
- obviously untrue negative thoughts.

Eating disorders

A possible association between CD and eating disorders such as anorexia nervosa and bulimia nervosa has received very little attention.

The causes of eating disorders are difficult to pinpoint, but biological, environmental and psychological factors are all likely to be involved. They are more common in younger women, but are not exclusively seen in this group.

You are more susceptible if you are anxious or depressed or have low self-esteem, or have experienced a stressful event. Some researchers think the Westernized ideal of thinness and the obsession with weight loss and celebrities or models can be a contributing factor. It would not be implausible that the weight gain in response to a GFD that many coeliacs experience could be a potential triggering issue for some women.

It is also possible that the great care that coeliacs need to take with their diets may, in vulnerable people, gradually slip towards hyper-obsessiveness, increasingly restricted diets and then anorexic behaviour.

Becoming obsessed with diet or size, being disturbed by minor weight gain, depression, social withdrawal, and excessive exercise are all signs of a problem.

Schizophrenia

Schizophrenia is a mental health illness, affecting thinking, feeling and behaviour. Age of onset is typically in the teenage or young adult years. Schizophrenia may involve disordered thoughts, delusions, hallucinations, apathy and lack of emotional response and interest.

A link between CD and schizophrenia is controversial, but has been the subject of speculation since the 1960s, when a researcher made the observation that it was rare in communities that consumed no wheat. The link is suspected by some, but if it exists the true nature of it remains unclear, although autoimmune mechanisms may be involved.

Studies have found around a third of those with schizophrenia have high levels of antibodies to gluten in their blood, and the basis for gluten as a trigger to some cases of schizophrenia is being explored.

Some people with schizophrenia may benefit from a GFD.

Self-help

So what can you do? Although there are plenty of ordinary people, specialists and groups who can help, there's one person who is undoubtedly the most important in your own emotional care and personal journey towards acceptance of your CD. You.

Positive learning

Learn everything you can about CD, and approach your fact-finding mission positively; your aim is to eliminate the anxiety which ignorance breeds.

If there is something that you do not understand about CD, a niggling query that is bothering you, then resolve to find the answer – if this book can't help, ask a health-care professional, or contact Coeliac UK. Getting on top of issues about which you're unsure is empowering.

Positive thinking

Remind yourself that your condition, despite being serious, is manageable. Focus on the positives: think of the foods that you can eat (there are hundreds), not those that you can't (there are only a handful); think of how your health will improve, not worsen, on a GFD.

Positive thinking also helps your self-esteem and self-confidence, vital when facing the gluten-containing world as a coeliac.

Exercise and activity

Good for you physically, but super on a mental level too. You don't have to join a gym. Don't run if you hate running. Merely resolving to take more walks is effective. Instead of focusing on the 'exercise' aspect, do something you love that involves activity and energy – such as amateur dramatics or DIY. Your body was designed to be active through living.

Fun and laughter

Humour is subjective, and what makes you laugh may make someone else scratch their head, but take part in fun activities, watch your favourite comedy shows to cheer you up, and share a joke with fellow coeliacs – whether it's over a dodgy coeliac tummy or the silly things that 'wheaties' (non-coeliacs) say.

Laughter is not the best medicine – nutritious GF food is – but it's still a very good one . . .

Pride

Why not? What's the alternative – shame?

Most people avoid certain foods. This can be for any number of reasons – ethical beliefs, religious beliefs, cultural beliefs, food allergies, food intolerances, unpalatability, health concerns. You don't eat gluten for a very good reason – and it's as valid as others' reasons for not eating peanuts, dairy or pork, for example. Have the same pride and confidence in your restriction as anyone else.

And if you don't want to always wear your 'coeliac hat'? That's OK too. You can be discreet – as long as it doesn't compromise your health.

Relaxation and breathing

Many people say they're unable to relax, but there is more to unwinding than just willing yourself to do so. Pampering – a hot bath, aromatherapy oils – can help, as can a massage from a willing partner. Meditation, prayer and chanting are deeply relaxing if they are right for you personally, as are forms of yoga and healing martial arts such as t'ai chi. Find what works for you, and remember that relaxation takes practice.

For instant stress relief if you're feeling uptight or nervous, try a technique of 'expanding' your peripheral vision. Find a point opposite you, just above eye-level, and keeping your eyes on that point, begin slowly to broaden your field of vision to notice more of what's on either side of the point, so that eventually you're paying attention to what is visible in the corners of your eyes. You should begin to feel your breathing moving lower in your chest, slowing down and becoming deeper, and your facial muscles relaxing. Very calming.

Indeed, learning to breathe correctly is of enormous value to stress relief: inhale deeply and slowly into the belly to the count of three, exhale evenly to the count of three, then pause for one – and repeat. Yogic breathing while seated and focusing on a lit candle is soothing.

Volunteering

Helping yourself by helping others can work wonders. Volunteering gives something back to the community, and will also strengthen your character and prove fulfilling.

Coeliac UK is always looking for volunteers to help with campaigning and research or to boost local support group membership and activities. The charity also supports members in organizing fundraising events. You could also get involved in educational activities: giving a demonstration of GF baking at your local school to kids, parents and teachers, for instance.

Volunteering can put you in touch with other coeliacs who can offer moral and practical support too.

Another option might be to volunteer to be a media 'case study': medical journalists often require these to illustrate articles in lifestyle magazines and newspaper health sections. CD is a popular subject, partly because it is so underdiagnosed, and there is a constant need for new case studies. They offer a chance to share your story: this can be therapeutic, and perhaps help readers to solve their own health predicaments. All that is usually required is a short telephone conversation with a journalist, and possibly a photograph.

Writing

Putting your anxieties and fears down on paper is an excellent way of clearing your head, unburdening yourself, understanding your problems and charting your emotional progress.

An alternative to keeping a private diary is keeping a public one – or a 'blog', which can be an online web diary of your experiences with CD and, well, anything you like. Coeliac blogs are very popular, and many coeliacs share their tips, recipes and thoughts online, and invite you to add comments. You may find your blog attracting attention from coeliacs worldwide. Comment on others' blogs and they're more likely to comment on yours.

Friends and family

The role of loved ones in your emotional care should never be underestimated. When you're first diagnosed, assess your support network and 'rally the troops' – your core group of partner, friends and family, who care for you and who you know can help you to come to terms with your condition.

The good guys

You need around you positive people who can offer practical advice and emotional support, who can lift your gloom and bring laughter into your life when you feel there is none, and who make you feel understood. The most valuable are the people who know your needs, the implications of your illness, who don't make you feel like a burden, who can act as your personal 'bodyguards' should you be tempted to cheat – and who don't make demands in return.

You also need people who are unafraid to give you difficult truths when they apply – to point out that you are foolishly taking risks with certain foods, or that you may benefit from seeking professional help with your mental health, for instance.

Shutting people out is a never-win situation. Most who care for you will want to help in any way they can, so don't be too proud to ask for practical help or a shoulder to cry on. You may feel you want to protect family members from the difficulties and implications of your CD, but, again, most prefer to be involved – even if it's just by helping you out with the GF groceries.

The not-so-good guys

Understand that not everyone you meet, work with or are friendly with will be helpful or supportive, often through ignorance not malice. Some people simply will not 'get' CD, refusing to believe that something as innocuous as wheat can make you so ill, and will insist that 'allergies are all in the mind' because an article they once read said so. Upsetting as this may be, this will probably always be the way to some extent, and arguing the case may not always prove fruitful, or make you feel better.

All friends have strengths and weaknesses, and much-valued confidantes may not necessarily be the right ones to turn to when you're suffering problems related to your CD; for instance:

- those who enjoy the 'fuss' of your CD, making an exaggerated issue of it at restaurants, for example;
- those who trivialize your condition and say you shouldn't take it so seriously; or
- those who 'hijack' your CD with their health problems less serious than your own.

Be aware of different people's reactions and be alert to those who make you feel worse. There's no shame in taking a step back if you need to. You must come first.

That said, remember too that people are more likely to be understanding and supportive if you demonstrate that you take your CD seriously. If you're a little reckless with label-reading or if you 'cheat' occasionally for a special occasion, people are understandably more likely to be sceptical.

Support groups

Occasionally, you may feel more comfortable seeking the support of strangers.

Charities

The Coeliac UK helpline (0845 305 2060) is staffed by knowledgeable people who can offer emotional as well as practical support. Other support lines of potential value include:

- Samaritans – 08457 909090

- Stress Anxiety Depression Helpline – 01622 717656
- beat (Eating Disorders Association) – 0845 634 1414

Even if you don't volunteer, taking part in local activities organized through Coeliac UK's support networks will relieve the isolation you may be feeling as a newly diagnosed coeliac.

Online support groups

Chat forums dedicated to those with CD – or other food-related sensitivities – can be supportive. People who live in secluded areas and feel isolated, those who are disabled, or single parents of young children, are among those who find these groups of particular value – but they can help anyone who perhaps is shy or has difficulty with face-to-face contact, and prefers the anonymity the internet offers.

Although groups can be encouraging, choose one with a knowledgeable moderator, who will remove suspect, offensive or dangerous postings. It is best to use them for matters such as emotional support, advice on food products, sharing recipes, tips on where to eat – rather than for medical advice.

Professional help

Sometimes, stubborn psychological problems need to be referred a step further.

Your GP

Doctors are your first port of call if you're suffering symptoms of stress, depression, anxiety or are concerned with other areas of your psychological health. Doctors are trained to see signs of emotional difficulties in their patients, and ideally placed to advise on possible private treatments or referrals. Do make use of your GP; many have good counselling skills and unburdening yourself to your GP may be all you need. He or she may also identify a need for a short course of anti-depressants, if relevant.

Your dietitian

If you're anxious about gluten avoidance or about nutrition, your dietitian can help fill the gaps in your knowledge and offer guidance and reassurance. Dietitians may also have a role to play in identifying and helping resolve possible eating disorders. Tempted to cheat? Missing bread? They can support and advise here too.

Your gastroenterologist

Your most complex queries can almost certainly be answered by your gastroenterologist. The more knowledge you demonstrate, and the more questions you ask of specialists, the more likely you will be given greater detail and reassurance.

If you feel burdened by not knowing whether or not you are improving on a GFD, a consultant can arrange a biopsy to check for gut recovery. If you feel tempted to cheat, a gastroenterologist can remind you of the seriousness of the damage you risk – that there's only so much recovery your gut can take, and that you're increasing your long-term risks of complications, such as osteoporosis and malignancies.

Life coaches

Increasingly popular, a life coach can help with motivation to change your lifestyle to benefit your health, give you confidence to talk to people about your dietary needs, and set goals towards making important changes fast, and less urgent ones gradually over time.

'Talking' therapists

If your doctor feels that you need more specialized help, referral for counselling or psychotherapy may be suggested. There are few specialists working in these fields in the NHS, so a private referral may be required.

There are few differences between the talking therapies, even though counselling sounds – and is – gentler and less demanding than psychotherapy. Both involve face-to-face meetings with a trained therapist to reach any number of end goals, depending entirely on the patient, such as the reduction of psychological distress and the promotion of emotional health.

Counsellors will listen to you, aim to identify with you and your dilemmas, help you to clarify them in your mind, and perhaps give advice – although generally their aim is to guide you to discover your own answers to your problems through carefully guided discussion. Counsellors can, for instance, help patients to cope and come to terms with difficult events like diagnosis.

Psychotherapists, of which there are many kinds, work similarly, but use more analytical approaches and explore difficulties in greater depth. They may work with those suffering from depression, anxiety and addictive behaviour disorders, those who are finding it difficult to adjust to their illness, and those whose condition is having an impact on many areas of their life.

Make sure you have an assessment session, and discontinue any therapy with a specialist with whom you feel uncomfortable – being at ease with your counsellor is vital. Remember too that counselling is not easy, or a magic wand: expect positive changes but not miracles. Some people approach therapy expecting their stresses to be entirely removed, but therapists will not do this: they will arm you with coping mechanisms, not seek to abolish all your responses.

Cognitive behaviour therapy (CBT)

CBT is an objective psychotherapeutic approach that is less interested in what caused your emotional or psychological difficulties, and more concerned with how you handle your dilemmas. It challenges negative thought patterns, helps you to identify and understand them, equips you with coping skills, and implements changes to unhelpful thinking or behaviour. The therapy is structured, practical and result-focused, unlike counselling, which usually involves 'freer' conversation and a greater rapport with the therapist.

CBT might be right for those looking for help with a specific issue. It is useful for depression, phobias or stress, for example, where the emphasis may be on cognition or thinking; while for eating disorders, predominantly behavioural issues will be tackled.

Hypnotherapy

This is a psychotherapy that uses hypnosis – a state of deep relaxation and heightened awareness, which makes the mind more receptive to positive suggestion. It can help those suffering from low self-esteem and anxiety, to name but two.

The road to acceptance

- Resolve to take positive action – learn to scrutinize labels, ask questions, learn everything you can about CD . . .
- Focus on everything positive – there are lots of new foods to enjoy, remember how much healthier you feel on the GFD, remind yourself you are on the road to recovery . . .
- Forgive yourself – if you make mistakes, if you feel grumpy, if you need some time to yourself . . .
- You are never alone – spend fun time with loved ones, talk to fellow coeliacs, call a support charity if you need one.

8

Practical issues

Coeliac disease (CD) may have an impact on other areas of your life as well.

Holidays and travel

You may feel nervous about travel, especially overseas, but by taking sensible measures there's no reason why you can't enjoy a trip anywhere, whether for business or pleasure.

Coeliac UK offers a number of resources, including leaflets on travelling to several dozen countries, with some useful phrases in translation, and there are a number of online sites offering recommendations. The charity carries advertising for many travel companies and hotels in its *Crossed Grain* magazine, and it can also recommend an insurance policy.

If travelling to Europe, apply for a European Health Insurance Card – see <www.ehic.org.uk> – before you travel. This card entitles you to medical treatment should you need it.

Research

Find out about your destination's food culture before you travel – some nations use little wheat (countries in the Far East), whereas others use it abundantly (most European nations).

If you're undecided where to go, bear in mind that although it may seem more logical to travel to a place where gluten grains are rarely used in the cuisine, in reality people in countries in which wheat or rye are common may be more likely to be coeliac-aware. Scandinavian nations, Ireland and Italy are good examples.

Holidaying in the UK or Ireland has obvious advantages. Many hotels are now promoting themselves as 'gluten-friendly' (or 'allergy-friendly') and actively encourage those with food sensitivities to stay.

Self-catering accommodation is an option, but if you're travelling somewhere rural check that you have easy access to a supermarket or store offering basic essentials.

Booking

If organizing your travel through an operator, let them know about your requirements – they may be able to make recommendations, and certainly try to accommodate you as much as possible.

When booking flights, specify that you need a gluten-free (GF) meal. Ask whether you can take GF food supplies in your luggage – a request that you may need to support with a medical note from your doctor. You may be able to increase your baggage allowance if you explain to the airline in advance. Consider packing toaster bags too.

Some countries have strict quarantine policies. For instance, Australia and New Zealand will allow you to bring certain GF staples in your luggage, but you must declare them and be prepared for them to be inspected on arrival.

Travelling

Have some snacks with you for whatever journey you undertake: finding GF options at motorway services, stations and airports is not always easy. Good options include homemade sandwiches made with GF bread, GF crackers, GF cereal bars, rice cakes, dried fruit and bananas.

Introduce yourself to cabin crew and remind them you requested a GF meal or snack when you booked.

Food labelling

There is no international agreement on the definition of 'gluten-free'.

The rest of the EU is subject to the same labelling legislation as the UK and Ireland. Here are some terms in various languages to look out for on food products:

- English: 'gluten-free', 'very low gluten'
- German: 'glutenfrei', 'sehr geringer glutengehalt'
- Dutch: 'glutenvrij', 'met zeer laag glutengehalte'
- French: 'sans gluten', 'très faible teneur en gluten'
- Italian: 'senza glutine', 'con contenuto di glutine molto basso'
- Spanish: 'exentos de gluten', 'contenido muy reducido de gluten'
- Portuguese: 'isento de glúten', 'teor muito baixo de glúten'.

For foods to be labelled 'gluten-free' in Australia and New Zealand they must contain 'no detectable gluten' (about 5 p.p.m. according to the best detection tests), which is considerably less than allowed elsewhere. Accordingly, you may find GF products there taste different.

According to the Canadian Celiac Association, 'Gluten-free in Canada means that the food does not contain wheat, spelt, kamut, rye, barley, oats or triticale, or any parts thereof . . . wheat starch is not permitted in a gluten-free diet.'

In the USA, the situation is subject to change. Wheat (but not yet gluten, or other gluten grains) must be declared on food labels, and the Food and Drug Administration is developing a definition for 'gluten-free', likely to be roughly in line with the EU's. Specialist products are of course available.

Outside those nations – in Africa and Asia, for instance – labelling may be less specific and more unreliable.

Remember that a particular brand or product that is safe in your home country may not be so in another nation.

Eating out

The same rules apply as at home. In countries where English isn't spoken you should still be able to find an English menu. Dietary cards explaining your requirements are available from some organizations if there is a language barrier issue, and may be worth ordering in advance.

Working life

Your CD should not hamper your working life or career choice – unless, perhaps, you wish to be a beer taster or restaurant reviewer! There are, for instance, plenty of successful athletes who are coeliacs.

Some jobs in which you may eat 'on the job' – pilot or flight attendant, for example – may require special provisions for your food, but as these are increasingly provided for passengers, again, there shouldn't be a special problem.

It is worth telling your employer that you are a coeliac. If you need to take time off for health appointments or if you've been 'glutened' and need to take a few days off work, your employer is likely to be more understanding if already aware of your condition.

The armed forces

The one exception is working in the armed forces. Those diagnosed with CD are not recruited because a guarantee to provide for a gluten-free diet (GFD) in the field or on operations is not feasible, according to the Ministry of Defence. Those diagnosed while serving will, where possible, be offered an alternative role or, if not, a medical discharge.

Beauty and grooming

Every day we wash, scrub, cleanse, moisturize, deodorize and condition parts of our body with a selection of gels, soaps, sprays, creams, colours and powders. Some of them may well use gluten-containing grains. How safe are they?

This is difficult to answer as no real research has been done on the subject. You will often hear quoted that a large proportion – up to 80 per cent – of what we apply to our skin is absorbed into the blood. This is exaggerated, and it varies depending on the product and the individual person. Even so, experts say that gluten is too large a molecule to pass through the skin barrier, and therefore should not pose a problem.

Lipsticks and lip balms are perhaps a more valid concern as they come into contact with the mouth, and trace amounts will be absorbed more readily and swallowed. Occasionally these products can contain ingredients derived from the gluten grains. All the major commercial brands of toothpastes and mouth washes avoid gluten-containing ingredients, and the same goes for most 'natural' brands of toothpaste, whose packaging may confirm this.

While the risk in the cases of lip products is unclear, but likely to be small, it is understandable that some coeliacs feel that they want to exclude gluten grains totally from their life regardless, and so may choose to adopt a no-wheat policy when it comes to their toiletries.

Product labelling

Although only food, and not cosmetic items, are bound by food allergen directives, and there are no specific rules for labelling gluten, ingredients must by law be listed on personal care products – either on the container or on the packaging. Cosmetics that are small and difficult to label clearly are partially exempt; instead, their ingredients should be displayed close to the item's point of sale or be available on a leaflet.

That said, botanicals are often in Latin and not English. Here are the ones that matter:

- Barley – *Hordeum* or *Hordeum vulgare*
- Oat – *Avena sativa*
- Rye – *Secale cereale*
- Wheat – *Triticum* or *Triticum vulgare*.

Grains tend to crop up in products of a thicker consistency, such as lip products, gels, creams and exfoliating scrubs, but occasionally deodorants contain wheat protein.

The notation [+/- . . .] indicates that the ingredient(s) listed in square brackets may or may not be present – the cosmetic equivalent of a 'may contain'.

Reactions to cosmetics

Reactions to cosmetics are common, and it is easy to assume that gluten may be a culprit, but it is unlikely.

Contact dermatitis, characterized by red itchy patches of skin, is the most common reaction. It is usually non-allergic and triggered by an irritant such as an abrasive or a detergent. The reaction is delayed not immediate, localized to the site of application, and usually caused by repeated exposure to the cosmetic, rather than one-off use. Those with eczema and very light-skinned people are more susceptible.

Allergic contact dermatitis is rarer. It is often caused by one or more of the many thousand fragrances found in bodycare products, but also by preservatives, ultraviolet filters and emulsifiers. Unlike irritant contact dermatitis, allergic contact dermatitis can spread beyond the site of application. Patch testing by a dermatologist can help identify culprits.

Immediate 'nettle' rashes are occasionally reported too, and it is known that these can be caused by hydrolysed wheat protein, among many other substances.

Other non-food exposures

Communion wafers

If you're a Roman Catholic, you may be concerned about holy communion. Roman Catholic doctrine specifies that the eucharistic wafers must be made from wheat and contain a trace of gluten. Other Christian churches aren't as strict, and allow wheat-free and GF bread.

Coeliac UK's website lists communion wafer suppliers in the UK, and suppliers are also noted in the Coeliac Society of Ireland's *Food List*. Those suitable for Roman Catholics are made from Codex wheat starch.

Pet food

Bear in mind that most dog and some cat food contains wheat as a filler. It's unlikely this will find its way into your mouth, but it is worth washing your hands carefully after handling and cleaning up carefully after your pet has fed.

Envelope gum

This is free from gluten.

9

Children and family

It is impossible for home life not to be impacted by coeliac disease (CD) when at least one member of the family has the condition. First-degree relatives of those with CD are ten times more likely to have it themselves, so it is natural to be concerned about all loved ones – especially children.

Pregnancy and birth

There is an increased risk of fertility difficulties as an undiagnosed coeliac, so if you are trying to conceive, are pregnant for the first time or are pregnant again following a miscarriage, you may be naturally nervous about carrying a child to term. Rest assured that a strict gluten-free diet (GFD) should soon normalize your fertility levels, and that there are no increased risks to you or your unborn child as a coeliac mum-to-be who adheres to the diet.

Before conceiving

If you're planning a pregnancy, discuss it with your health-care advisers. It may not be advisable to try to conceive soon after your diagnosis if you have a compromised nutritional status.

Your intake and levels of folic acid (folate) are key. You may be deficient in this B vitamin, and all women are advised to supplement with 400 micrograms of folic acid daily as soon as they stop using contraception, and to increase their intake of folic acid with, for example, green vegetables. Women with CD may need a little more, so speak to your dietitian. Folic acid helps to prevent neural-tube disorders such as spina bifida in your unborn child.

During pregnancy

General healthy eating guidelines, many outlined in Chapter 5, apply to all mothers-to-be too: at least five portions of fruit and vegetables daily, lots of gluten-free (GF) starches and grains, plenty of fluids, moderate caffeine intake – but no alcohol.

Calcium intake is particularly important in pregnancy, especially in coeliac mums, and low-fat dairy products are recommended.

Similarly, iron intake, too, is key – meats, fish, eggs and pulses supply iron, as well as vital protein. Only supplement with iron on medical advice.

Try GF crackers or rice cakes if you need to nibble something to help with morning sickness.

The Department of Health advises all women to avoid certain foods in pregnancy:

- Raw and partially cooked eggs
- Raw shellfish and meats
- Blue-veined and soft-ripened cheeses
- Pâtés
- Shark, marlin and swordfish
- Liver and liver products.

Your prescription entitlement increases in the third trimester of your pregnancy, so take advantage of this and review the foods you need with your dietitian.

Childbirth

There are no particular considerations for coeliac women in childbirth, although some studies suggest that giving birth naturally rather than via Caesarean section decreases the likelihood of your child developing CD in later life.

Early feeding

Exclusive breastfeeding in the first six months is the best thing you can do for your child's health – and research suggests that this can offer some protection against the development of CD later on. You are entitled to four additional units of prescription GF food when breastfeeding.

Formula milk provides all the nutrition your baby needs, and all is GF.

Weaning

Some babies aren't satisfied with a milk-only diet until six months, and may need to start solids a little sooner – but never before four months. Discuss this with your midwife or health-care adviser.

Gluten should not be introduced into any baby's diet before six months, but there appear to be no benefits for delaying it any longer than this. Coeliac UK advises that once a baby is established on solids, gluten should be given regularly, since CD can only be diagnosed once gluten is established in the diet. Should symptoms occur (see p. 2), they are usually very obvious at this young age.

Extended breastfeeding during weaning also appears to be protective, although whether this delays or prevents the onset of CD is still being examined.

The weaning advice to babies at higher risk of CD is subject to change, owing to ongoing studies in this area, so always take your definitive advice from Coeliac UK or your health-care advisers.

Children and CD

If you have a child who is newly diagnosed with CD you will feel a mix of emotions: protective, anxious, fearful, relieved. It may be some consolation to know that children are tough little things who adapt superbly to the new requirements – possibly because they won't consider their diet to be a priority in their lives at that age. At a time when they're still growing and developing, lasting damage caused by poor absorption of food and malnutrition is also unlikely.

It's generally good advice to focus on the present – do what you need to do *now* – and cross certain bridges when you come to them.

You will have access to a specialist paediatric dietitian if your child is diagnosed with CD, who will be best placed to advise on any nutritional concerns. There are no specific recommendations for coeliac children, but the dietitian will ensure that you understand the need for a healthy GFD and an adequate intake of such minerals as calcium and iron. Some children may have anaemia on diagnosis, so this will be addressed.

If diagnosed in infancy, your child may not have been exposed to too many gluten-containing foods, and so he or she may not be too concerned with (or even notice) the sudden change in diet. Your child may, though, have made the connection with having felt sick and the previous diet, and so may be more aware than you think. You will certainly need to talk to your child at some point – the sooner the better – and this really depends on the level of maturity and when you feel your child is ready. Here are some tips:

- The name 'coeliac disease' features the word 'disease' right there in the name: this can alarm children, so it may be better to talk in terms of a 'poorly tummy' caused by gluten.
- Get children involved in food selection and cooking as soon as possible. Learning about GF foods can take place during supermarket shops, meal preparation and outings to restaurants – let them try

to choose foods and order their own meals, for instance, and teach them to articulate their requirements to waiting staff.

- Introduce them to new foods regularly – including the unusual ones. Quinoa was the ancient grain of the Incas – build a story, a history lesson, around it to appeal to them.
- Teach them how to decline food. 'No thank you' may be better than 'I can't eat that.' Teach them that what they put into their bodies is up to them, and there's no obligation to eat something they don't like, even if GF, or if a relative has 'made it specially'.
- Don't overwhelm children with information at first – issues such as cross-contamination need to be conveyed eventually, but this is something you can manage on their behalf at first.
- Teach them about labelling gradually – the Crossed Grain symbol is one that they can learn to look out for to help 'break in' to the subject.
- Be positive and upbeat about the situation – your child will pick up on it if you display fretfulness about it. The GFD is absolutely manageable and it's important to convey this to your child.
- Explain CD to other children in the family too. Siblings need to understand the situation and feel involved in the family's care of the coeliac child.
- All kids deserve a treat or reward from time to time, but don't give a coeliac child two treats where you might only give a non-coeliac child one – it's easy to feel you have to offer an extra 'bonus' snack as compensation for having the condition, but ultimately it's not good for the child or the child's tummy.
- If the household is not going GF, it may be helpful to use 'safe' stickers to highlight coeliac-friendly food – you can turn this into an educational game.
- Coeliac UK publishes very useful booklets for parents and carers: *Getting Started*, *Out and About* and *Me and My Tummy*.

Nursery and school

Sending your coeliac child to school can be nerve-racking because suddenly he or she will be under someone else's care and can potentially be exposed to risky foods such as crisps and wheat snacks.

Coeliac UK can send you a parents' information pack, with information on how to inform your child's nursery or school about the condition. Conveying key information to staff is vital, and Coeliac UK offers a draft letter on its website. You should explain what CD is, that your child is on a GFD, where gluten is found and what your child cannot eat.

You will also need to broach the issue of school lunches, and whether your child will be bringing his or her own, or whether catering systems are in place to cater or potentially cater for your child (schools aren't obliged to provide GF meals – but a meeting with the head of catering can be productive). You may feel happier, at least initially, providing a GF packed lunch, in which case you will need to check how closely children are supervised to prevent them swapping foods.

Autism and CD

According to the National Institute for Health and Clinical Excellence: 'There is no conclusive evidence on the prevalence of coeliac disease in people with autism. Anecdotally, higher rates of coeliac disease are seen in people with autism, and when diagnosed, adherence to a gluten-free diet improves both gastrointestinal symptoms and behavioural problems. Research is needed to determine the prevalence of coeliac disease in people with autism and whether any behavioural problems improve following diagnosis.'

Social events

With regard to after-school activities and children's social clubs, communication is key. Those in charge will be understanding and appreciate the need for vigilance if you convey the seriousness of CD. In situations where children may be given treats, it helps if you supply adults in charge with some GF treats in advance as a standby.

Parties present a bigger problem, as you can't expect other children's parents to serve GF food exclusively. Speak with them well in advance, in person not on the phone, and offer to supply a GF replacement party parcel for your child, clearly labelled, or to provide a GF cake for the birthday child.

Accept that mistakes will happen, and your child may get a little sick. Never punish your child for this. Remember that being 'glutened' may lay your child low for a while, but he or she will get better. Make the best of the bad situation and review the importance of not swapping food or thoughtlessly popping treats into the mouth. Your child is likely to remember the effects of the accident, and will instinctively be more careful in future.

Teenagers and CD

Teenagers are rarely diagnosed with CD, so any teenagers with the condition are likely to have had it for some years. At this age, they should be well established on the GFD and understand how to manage their lifestyle. Nevertheless, this is the time during which some teens can get a bit reckless with their diet, possibly as a minor act of rebellion that's sometimes characteristic of this stage of life.

Some teenagers may be curious – 'What does wheat taste like? I wonder if a "real" pizza tastes better than the one I have to eat?' Some succumb to peer pressure – boys especially may be 'dared' to consume a harmful food. Some just get complacent. They may have been well for years. Boys may see themselves as strong and immortal, about to become men, and may feel it isn't macho to 'fuss' about food. They may take risks, and may hide it from you, possibly because they don't want you to worry.

It's understandable. Teens want to fit in, not stand out, and they don't want to have to ask to see a label when their mates offer them a sweet from a bag.

The problem with risk-taking is that they may not experience any symptoms. It's a curious fact about the growing teenage coeliac body that it appears adept at not producing overt symptoms of gluten consumption – which is possibly why few are diagnosed at this time. Your son or daughter may feel perfectly well, which could justify and excuse the gluten consumption in his or her mind.

It's worth watching out for any change in health or behaviour, and talking to your teen regularly about the GFD in a non-judgemental or castigating way, reminding him or her that damage can be silent, and reiterating the importance of the diet.

But don't get paranoid: many teens manage their GFD and lifestyle with exceptional maturity.

University

Try not to worry or make too much of a fuss. Equip them with practical things before they set off – toaster bags, some GF supplies, a GF cookbook, their own bread board and biscuit tin. Ensure that they know that they have to communicate their CD to flatmates and fellow students and university caterers. It's pointless to advise most young adults not to drink – but do warn them to stay away from beers. A GF food parcel after a few weeks will be warmly received.

10

Staying well

Coeliac disease (CD) is a lifelong condition and – at least for the fore-seeable future – incurable. While the advice in earlier chapters has been mostly focused on getting you or your child better, you need to be aware of how to best stay that way – for life – and overcome any stumbling blocks along the way.

Dietary compliance

It's worth repeating that a strict gluten-free diet (GFD) is the most important strategy for ongoing health and well-being.

Compliance among coeliacs is not always good, and surveys suggest that anywhere between only 45 per cent and 90 per cent stick to the GFD. More at risk of lapses are those who experienced few or only mild symptoms prior to diagnosis.

You should not be reassured by any thoughts of 'safety in numbers' from those percentages – all coeliacs who stray run increased risks of associated short-term and long-term health problems, including abdominal symptoms, poor pregnancy outcomes, nutrient deficiencies and reduced bone mineral density – and possibly other autoimmune diseases.

There may be a number of contributory factors to non-compliance:

- Inconvenience – obtaining safe food is more time-consuming, and scanning the sometimes tiny print on food labels can be frustrating.
- Cost – specialist gluten-free (GF) food is often more expensive.
- Unpalatability – you may miss ordinary bread and pasta, for example, and dislike their replacements.
- Social issues – peer pressure, not wishing to appear different or 'make a fuss'.
- Denial – those with no or few symptoms prior to diagnosis may feel they can 'get away' with consuming occasional gluten as they con-sider themselves healthy.
- Symptom-free lapses – failure to experience any abdominal side-effects with gluten intake may reinforce the idea that occasional cheats are OK.

Do resist any urge to cheat. Understand that temptation is likely to come from many sources, and will always crop up from time to time. Be prepared for situations where temptation may arise, and remember that all foods have a GF version these days, so you don't need to sacrifice a particular type of food. It's not the bland taste of gluten you're missing or craving – just the familiar one of that sweet or savoury something in which it is found.

Being 'glutened'

Despite your best intentions, accidents will happen, and you will probably consume some gluten at some point during your GFD, be it through food mistakenly served to you, through cross-contamination or through personal error. Never punish yourself for this. It happens to all.

In some cases, symptoms may be mild; in others, very severe. The usual symptom is diarrhoea, often starting the day after, and continuing ill health – perhaps headaches, stomach pain, lethargy – for up to a week or longer. Sometimes the symptoms begin extremely quickly after ingestion. It varies.

Don't make yourself sick if you realize what's happened – this can be dangerous. The deed is done. Rest, eat plain food, perhaps avoiding dairy products for a while, and drink lots of fluids if you have diarrhoea – and ideally a diarrhoea replacement drink too.

There are some digestive enzymes on the market whose manufacturers claim can help with the digestion of gluten and that some coeliacs take when they've inadvertently consumed gluten. These may help to reduce symptoms caused by accidental exposure, but there is no evidence they work and any effects may only be psychological. These enzymes should *never* be used as a means by which to cheat on the GFD.

Remember that, just like anyone else, coeliacs are prone to upset tummies for other reasons, such as food poisoning, eating rich and spicy foods, consuming too much alcohol or even eating something new that just didn't agree with them. If you do feel 'glutened', it may not always have been gluten.

Ongoing symptoms

The gut can take up to two years to heal, so don't be surprised if you experience occasional symptoms during the recovery period.

With regard to ongoing symptoms, the most common reason is non-compliance with the GFD, either deliberately or unknowingly. In the latter case, try to examine whether gluten could be sneaking into your diet, perhaps over a meeting with your dietitian:

- Are you reading and re-reading labels carefully to make sure foods are GF?
- Have you written a detailed food diary and gone through it with your dietitian to identify possible problems?
- Have you ruled out any cross-contamination possibilities from your kitchen – or other sources?
- Are you consuming a lot of barley malt flavouring or extract?
- Could you be consuming contaminated oats? Or could you be one of the few coeliacs sensitive to even GF oats?
- Are you following a diet high in prescription products made with Codex wheat starch – to which some coeliacs may be sensitive?

The question of a 'safe' level of gluten consumption in coeliacs remains unanswered. Studies suggest that a long-term daily intake of 10–50mg of gluten could trigger damage to the gut lining – 500g of GF bread or pasta at 20 p.p.m. would equate to the lowest level (i.e. 10mg). Note, though, that this is the most sensitive end of the scale, that it is unlikely you will consume half a kilogram of GF replacement products a day, and most of those foods will contain less than 20 p.p.m. of gluten anyway. It may be more of an issue with 'very low gluten' foods, however.

Note too that reactions to Codex wheat starch may not be quite what they seem (see p. 96).

Food intolerances

Other food intolerances, perhaps temporary ones, may also be an issue in CD, and may be worth considering if accidental gluten intake has been ruled out. The symptoms are usually digestive-based, and similar to those found in undiagnosed CD and irritable bowel syndrome.

Lactose intolerance

Lactose is the type of sugar found in fresh milk, and it is present to a lesser extent in all other foods made from milk, such as yoghurts and cheeses. Our usual intake is through cows' milk products, but the milk of all mammals, including goats and sheep, also contains lactose.

The digestive enzyme that breaks down lactose is called lactase, and this is produced in the tips of the villi that line the gut. Damage to your gut lining caused by CD may mean that your body's ability to produce lactase is hampered, and so the lactose you consume remains undigested. Undigested lactose in the gut attracts water and passes rapidly through the system to the large bowel, where bacteria ferment it, forming waste gases. This process is responsible for the main unpleasant symptoms of lactose intolerance, such as bloating, abdominal pain, flatulence and frothy diarrhoea, typically half an hour or more after the consumption of dairy products.

If there is any doubt, a simple test is available from your doctor or dietitian, which measures hydrogen levels in your breath following consumption of milk.

If lactose intolerance is confirmed, you will need to avoid milk and ice cream, and perhaps other dairy products, depending on your sensitivity, which you'll usually be able to gauge by trial and error. Yoghurts and cheeses are lower in lactose and may be tolerated well. It is better to eat these foods with other foods, rather than on an empty stomach, as they will be better tolerated.

Low-lactose milks and other dairy products are now available on the market, and there are plenty of dairy-free milks and related products too.

Alternative sources of calcium (see p. 56) must be included in the diet if lactose intolerance is severe enough to warrant a dairy-free or reduced-diary diet.

As one of the key allergens, milk must be mentioned on food labelling. Many 'free-from' products are dairy-free, but this may not be flagged as prominently as their gluten-free or wheat-free status.

Lactose intolerance caused by CD is usually temporary, but in some cases may last for a year or more even on the GFD, until the gut heals sufficiently and the ability to produce lactase is restored. You can try to increase or reintroduce lactose-containing foods gradually over time, perhaps under the guidance of your dietitian, and this in itself may help to 'retrain' your system to accept lactose again.

Other sugar intolerances

There are other sugar intolerances. These are given considerably less attention in the medical literature and appear to be under-recognized.

Fructose intolerance or malabsorption

Like glucose, fructose is a type of simple sugar. Unlike glucose, though, it is poorly absorbed by the body, and those with digestive problems such as irritable bowel syndrome or CD may have greater difficulty than others absorbing it. In CD, this may be caused by damage to the villi. When this happens, the fructose passes through to the colon, where it is fermented. The resulting symptoms are similar to those encountered in lactose intolerance, and again a hydrogen breath test may help to identify the intolerance.

There are several sources of fructose in the diet:

- Many fruits (e.g. apples, grapes, melons, pears) and dried fruit
- Many fruit juices and fruit juice concentrates
- Table sugar (i.e. sucrose – in which fructose is bound with glucose)
- More complex fructose sugars called fructans, such as the prebiotics fructo-oligosaccharides and inulin – found in wheat starch, onion, leek, artichokes and asparagus
- Corn syrup and high-fructose corn syrup
- Honey, treacle, coconut milk and coconut cream.

Malabsorption of polyols (sugar alcohols)

Not alcoholic in the usual sense, the sugar alcohols, or polyols, include sorbitol, maltitol, mannitol, xylitol and isomalt. They are used as sweeteners in the food industry, and they only weakly raise blood sugar levels. This is due to humans' inability to absorb them efficiently.

Because of this low absorbability, the sugar alcohols may trigger symptoms similar to those that can be triggered by fructose and lactose.

They tend to be used in slimming drinks and diet foods, chewing gum, low-sugar soft drinks and diabetic foods. But they are naturally found in some fruits and their juices, too: for instance, sorbitol is found in apples, pears and some stone fruit (e.g. plums), and xylitol in berries.

The low-FODMAP diet

FODMAP stands for 'fermentable oligo-, di- and mono-saccharides and polyols' – which essentially refers to most of the types of sugars mentioned above that may be poorly absorbed, especially by coeliacs, and that may be therefore implicated in ongoing symptoms in some people with CD. A diet low in FODMAPs may be worth a try in certain circumstances, but you *must* discuss this with your dietitian and only attempt it under dietetic guidance and support.

Wheat and other intolerances

You already react severely to the gluten in wheat – but a minority of coeliacs may also react in a different way to other parts of wheat, such as the carbohydrate or fibre. On a GFD, the most likely exposure to this is via Codex wheat starch in 'free-from' foods. The trace levels of gluten in these products do seem to affect some very sensitive coeliacs, but other coeliacs who feel that they get symptoms from Codex wheat starch may be reacting to the starch itself. This can be very tricky to unpick. It may be worth trying a wheat-free diet for a while – some pre-scription foods and many supermarket 'free-from' foods are wheat-free – but again try it only under the guidance of a dietitian, never alone.

Intolerance to Codex wheat starch may theoretically be related to its fructans content (see p. 95).

Other intolerances – to foods such as soya and egg – are possible but less common.

Exclusion or elimination diets

Intolerances to wheat and other natural foods cannot be tested for with the hydrogen breath test as sugar intolerances can be, and there are no reliable tests for them. (The tests described on p. 19 are either unscien-tific or considered unproven.)

The only way to diagnose one is through an exclusion diet. This is a diagnostic test diet from which suspect foods are first removed for several weeks. If symptoms persist, it's either a psychological food aver-sion or not food-related at all. If symptoms clear, a food intolerance can be diagnosed and the reintroduction phase can begin, where foods are individually and gradually brought back into the diet in order to monitor reactions. The reintroduction of a food followed by the return of symptoms is considered indicative of an intolerance to it.

Many intolerances are identified in this way, but other people re-introduce all foods without problems – a change of diet can sometimes be all that's needed to clear up symptoms.

Willpower and patience are needed to adhere to the diet, but it is quite effective in diagnosing a problem food. You must never attempt it without the guidance and close supervision of a dietitian, not least because the results can be so difficult to interpret and nutritional advice will be needed.

In practice, your dietitian is unlikely to want to tinker with your diet in this way, at least not soon after diagnosis, and the priority will be to make sure that you are successfully established on a nutritious GFD before looking at other concerns.

Ongoing problems: other possibilities

There are a few other causes of persistent tummy troubles.

Irritable bowel syndrome

This is common in the general population, and can co-exist with CD. Often it is linked to stress.

Around 10 per cent of coeliacs who don't respond to the GFD may have underlying irritable bowel too, and it is possible that the symptoms they were experiencing that led to their coeliac diagnosis may actually have been caused by undiagnosed irritable bowel syndrome, while their CD was 'silent' all along.

Irritable bowel syndrome can be diagnosed only by your doctor. Your doctor or dietitian may advise adjustments to your fibre intake, perhaps reducing your intake of insoluble fibre (e.g. whole grains) and increasing your intake of soluble fibre (e.g. vegetables, oats). Other dietary modifications may help, but what works for one person will not work for another, so advice must be individualized.

Some general tips are to eat at regular intervals and not to skip meals, and to reduce intake of caffeinated, fizzy or alcoholic drinks.

Anti-spasmodic medication may be recommended, and relaxation therapy or hypnotherapy has been shown to help with irritable bowel syndrome.

Small intestinal bacterial overgrowth

Small intestinal bacterial overgrowth (SIBO), or small bowel bacterial overgrowth (SBBO), is a condition in which there is an excess of bacteria in the small intestine, leading to symptoms of diarrhoea, wind, pain and bloating. According to the British Society of Gastroenterology, it is underdiagnosed in the population, and may well occur in some coeliac patients who have ongoing problems despite a GFD.

It can be diagnosed with a breath test, and antibiotics are the usual course of treatment. Taking probiotics (see p. 61) may offer some benefits in addition, as may reducing your sugar intake, but do check with your doctor first.

Poor diet

Is your GFD healthy? It's an important question, one which you should ask yourself honestly. It can be so tempting to comfort eat after a coeliac diagnosis, but your diet needs to be balanced in order to encourage recovery at a time when your gut lining is trying to heal. You need lots of nourishing and nutrient-dense foods. Try to avoid sweet foods, which could lead to problems with sugar absorption, as discussed above. See p. 52 for healthy eating advice.

Pancreatic insufficiency

This is the inability to properly digest food as a result of poor production of digestive enzymes by the pancreas. It may result in poor absorption, and the consequent symptoms. It has been proposed as a not uncommon problem in CD patients with persistent symptoms. It is more likely if you also have type 1 diabetes. It can be diagnosed via a stool test, and the treatment is enzyme supplementation.

Mistaken diagnosis

It is possible for people to be misdiagnosed with CD when they don't have it, but this is rare these days, owing to advances in diagnostic procedures and awareness.

Aftercare

It's vital that you accept a lifetime of follow-up care, as research shows that it helps you to stick to a GFD. It also allows you to discuss and hopefully resolve the possible problems discussed above. That said, a lack of local resources may mean that you may not receive the ideal level of aftercare. See your doctor or speak to Coeliac UK if this is a problem in your area or if you are left largely to manage on your own.

Your dietitian

Ideally, you should have subsequent appointments with your dietitian or paediatric dietitian every three months in the first year following diagnosis. This is helpful for reviewing your progress and your understanding of the GFD, for untangling any sticking points and for addressing any ongoing nutritional problems. Your dietitian can also help with any struggles to maintain your GFD and ongoing symptoms – perhaps by checking your understanding of food labelling or by ordering further tests.

Children must be closely monitored and examined to ensure that their development and growth progress normally. A dietary assessment by a paediatric dietitian can help to identify nutritional deficiencies and any need for supplements.

Your GP

Use your GP as an ongoing source of health advice and support – he or she can help with your prescriptions, with arranging or performing further tests and with recommending vaccinations and so on – but may also conduct your annual follow-up and assessment.

Your gastroenterologist

Patients obviously want access to their gut specialists, and they are often best placed to answer questions specifically related to gut health concerns. A paediatrician may be involved in the care of your child. Reviews at your gastroenterology clinic after three and six months are recommended.

Follow-up tests

There are several follow-up tests that you may need.

Blood tests

A full blood count and a check of nutrient levels should ideally be performed every year, and more regularly under particular circumstances.

Coeliac antibody tests (i.e. a tTG test) may be repeated as regularly, to check that the levels of antibodies to tissue transglutaminase have reduced. In children, it is recommended that these tests be performed after six months of a GFD. In practice, children dislike giving blood, and if the consultant believes recovery is strong after several years, blood tests may not always be performed unless there is a specific concern.

Serious complications

These are very rare in CD, but still do occur.

Refractory CD is CD in which the gut does not heal on a strict GFD. One form can be treated with corticosteroids and the prognosis is good, but the second form is more serious, and lymphoma (cancer) of the intestine usually follows, which has a poor prognosis.

There is a slightly increased chance of other malignancies of the gastrointestinal tract among newly diagnosed patients with CD, but once established on the GFD for several years, the risk becomes equivalent to that of a non-coeliac. The risk of cancer is much lower than previously thought, and is very small, especially when adhering to a strict GFD.

DEXA bone scan

Those with abnormal bone density should be reassessed every three years. Children are unlikely to require a DEXA scan.

Endoscopy and biopsy

When there are continued symptoms and other possibilities have been ruled out, a repeat biopsy may be advised in order to check whether there has been improvement in the health of the mucosa. Another case may be made for a repeat biopsy if the initial diagnosis was not 100 per cent secure. You might want one yourself, to confirm that the effort of the strict GFD you are undertaking is reaping rewards in gut health.

There is some disagreement over the value of a repeat biopsy, so this will depend very much on your personal circumstances and the view of your consultant.

In cases where the reintroduction of GF oats into the diet following improvement results in the return of symptoms, the British Society of Gastroenterology advises that it may be worth considering a repeat biopsy to examine the villi.

In children diagnosed before the age of two, a gluten challenge followed by a biopsy may be recommended at some point, typically around the age of six or seven years, to confirm a questionable initial diagnosis. In a gluten challenge, 10 grams of gluten must be reintroduced into the diet every day for at least six weeks prior to the biopsy.

Other tests

Liver or thyroid function tests may be appropriate.

11

The outlook

Most in the professional coeliac community believe that alternatives to the gluten-free diet (GFD) are urgently needed, largely because the diet is expensive and difficult and because compliance with it sometimes poor. Further, coeliac disease (CD) is on the rise worldwide and there is concern that this will increasingly burden health-care providers, adding to the demands placed upon them by low diagnosis rates.

Future treatments

There are four possibilities:

1 Treatments that work in addition to a GFD
2 Treatments that minimize possible health effects of hidden, trace or accidentally consumed gluten in the GFD
3 Treatments that allow moderate gluten consumption
4 Treatments that replace the GFD and allow a regular diet.

There are various treatments being proposed, developed and trialled at the beginning of the second decade of the new millennium, and some are considered below. It has been speculated that it may not be until 2020 that one or more become widely available commercially. Some may fail at trial stage if, for instance, unacceptable side-effects should be encountered, but even a single viable one could transform lives – if only by offering greater peace of mind and reduced risks of the usual effects of cross-contamination when dining out.

Vaccine therapy

Of the many thousands of protein parts (peptides) found in gluten, the bulk of the immune response activated in CD is caused by just three, and it is these three that are most toxic to coeliacs. From this starting point, scientists at the Walter and Eliza Hall Institute in Melbourne, Australia, led by Dr Robert Anderson, have developed a potential vaccine, Nexvax2, which has been synthesized to work by 'introducing' these fragments of gluten to the immune system of coeliacs in a particular way, 're-educating' them to tolerate the protein and not to react inappropriately. It has the potential to treat 80 per cent of those with CD, say the researchers.

Enzyme therapy

Alvine Pharmaceuticals' enzyme treatment, ALV003, is a therapy that helps to break down the toxic fragments of gluten in the stomach when taken before a gluten-containing meal.

Other protein enzymes – called proteases – may also have potential in the development of new 'free-from' foods, serving to 'pre-digest' gluten in order to formulate more palatable products.

Helminthic therapy

Not for the squeamish, this involves inoculating CD patients with a harmless hookworm to interfere with immune responses and alter responsivity to gluten. This is based on the idea that our sterile Western modes of living and antibiotic-rich medicine cabinets, which have eradicated intestinal parasitic worms from our bodies, have detrimentally affected our immune responses, increasing the tendency towards autoimmune conditions such as CD. Kept 'distracted' by these parasites, the immune system ought to ignore the mistaken 'threat' of gluten, holds the theory.

Other therapies

AT-1001 (larazotide) is a promising drug that blocks the action of zonulin, a protein that 'unlocks' the intestinal barrier and increases the gut's permeability, or leakiness. Those with autoimmune disease produce higher levels of zonulin. Alba Therapeutics Corporation in the US, founded by Dr Alessio Fasano of the University of Maryland Center for Celiac Research, has conducted promising trials.

Meanwhile, CCX282-B is an anti-inflammatory drug that works by restricting the movement of certain immune cells – which trigger the coeliac response – from the bloodstream into the gut wall.

Prevention

The maxim certainly applies: prevention is clearly better than cure.

Probiotics

It has been theorized that the balance of bacteria that we all carry naturally in our digestive system could have relevance in the development of CD, given that many people show the first symptoms of the disease when this balance has been upset – following gastrointestinal surgery, for instance, or food poisoning. Correcting this upset with the introduction of certain probiotics could lead to a potential preventative treatment.

Optimized gluten introduction

When is the best time to introduce gluten into an at-risk baby's diet in order to induce tolerance? A few studies have looked at this vital unanswered question, and results appear to indicate that there may be a 'window of opportunity' at between four and six months that may be ideal. Further prospective studies are ongoing. The quantity of gluten given at various stages may also be a factor.

An Italian trial, though, found that delayed introduction to one year was associated with a considerably lower risk of developing CD after five years than introduction at six months – although further follow-up for many years will be needed as this may not indicate a different lifetime prevalence.

Other vaccination

Children genetically predisposed to CD appear more likely to develop the disease after a rotavirus infection – opening the possibility that an anti-rotavirus vaccine may offer some protection in a subset of infants.

New wheats and breads

Genetic modification of wheat is potentially revolutionary. Some researchers have suggested it may be possible to 'breed out' the toxic elements of gluten, rendering a wheat safe for consumption by all.

Older and more 'natural' forms of wheat may also be exploited, as these are known to be less toxic than modern types of wheat, which have been bred for their rich gluten content and associated culinary properties.

The use of *Lactobacillus* bacteria in sourdough bread has also aroused interest: it appears in pilot studies that these bacteria can break down toxic gluten peptides, rendering the bread safe, or at least safer, but further studies are needed.

Diagnosis

The debate over whether a biopsy should be required to diagnose CD remains active. Some feel that a combination of increasingly reliable blood tests and strong clinical symptoms should be sufficient in at least a proportion of cases; others feel that a biopsy should remain mandatory.

New and improved tests could eventually make the question redundant. A test for antibodies to the three peptides found to be most toxic is one possible avenue. Another test to detect certain proteins in the urine – also a future possibility – would be even less invasive.

CD-Medics is a European project developing a point-of-care test to measure both coeliac antibodies and genes.

Diagnostic criteria are likely to remain in flux for some time, and revisions to recommendations will be inevitable.

Screening

Screening is a strategy used to look for disease where no signs of it exist. Screening for CD in at-risk groups (e.g. first-degree relatives of patients) is recommended, and this 'case-finding' can be highly effective. But should universal screening – that is, screening of the whole population for CD – be implemented? It is a future possibility, with some arguing that a coeliac test should become as routine as a cholesterol test.

Controversies

Inevitably in such an active field, there is much disagreement and debate.

Some experts feel that research would be better geared towards the development of more innovative gluten-free (GF) foods – not drugs and vaccines. Some coeliacs, equally, are quite happy to live a GF lifestyle, aren't interested in a future of wheat reintroduction, but would welcome wider and more affordable choices from the supermarket.

The issue of screening is widely debated. Obviously, this would help to diagnose coeliacs and find the missing millions we know are out there, but on the other hand, there is the moral concern that it would 'impose' disease on people who may consider themselves healthy and not wish to know otherwise. The burden on health care must also be considered.

Genetic modification of wheat is obviously controversial.

Moving forward

Never before has CD been the subject of so much attention, or been so visible in the public domain. It is impossible to predict what its future may be, or what implications this will have for those with the disease or at risk of developing it.

What is indisputable is that its conspicuous profile can only be regarded as a very good thing indeed.

Further reading

Books

Allen, Darina, and Kearney, Rosemary, *Healthy Gluten-free Eating*, Kyle Cathie, 2009

Baic, Sue, Denby, Nigel, and Korn, Danna, *Living Gluten-free for Dummies*, John Wiley and Sons, 2007

Gazzola, Alex, *Living with Food Intolerance*, Sheldon Press, 2005

Holmes, Geoffrey, Catassi, Carlo, and Fasano, Alessio, *Fast Facts: Celiac Disease*, Health Press, 2009

Howdle, Peter, *Your Guide to Coeliac Disease*, Hodder Education, 2007

Humphries, Carolyn, *Gluten-free Bread and Cakes from Your Breadmaker*, W. Foulsham, 2009

James Ahern, Shauna, *Gluten-Free Girl*, John Wiley and Sons, 2009

Koeller, Kim, and La France, Robert, *Let's Eat Out with Celiac/Coeliac and Food Allergies!* R&R Publishing, 2009

Rabinovich, Adriana, *The Gluten-free Cookbook for Kids*, Vermilion, 2009

Skypala, Isabel, and Venter, Carina, *Food Hypersensitivity*, Wiley-Blackwell, 2009

Vickery, Phil, *Seriously Good! Gluten-free Baking*, Kyle Cathie, 2010

Vickery, Phil, *Seriously Good! Gluten-free Cooking*, Kyle Cathie, 2009

Print magazines

Allergic Living (Canada): www.allergicliving.com
Gluten-free Living (USA): www.glutenfreeliving.com
Living Without (USA): www.livingwithout.com

Webzines and blogs

Alex Gazzola's blog: www.foodallergyandintolerance.blogspot.com
Celiac.com (USA): www.celiac.com
Celiac-Disease.com (USA): www.celiac-disease.com
FoodsMatter.com: www.foodsmatter.com
GFLiving (Ireland): www.gfliving.com
The Gluten Free Blog: www.gluten-free-blog.com
Gluten-free Girl and The Chef (USA): www.glutenfreegirl.blogspot.com
The Intolerant Gourmet: www.theintolerantgourmet.com

Useful addresses

Coeliac charities

Coeliac UK
Third Floor, Apollo Centre
Desborough Road
High Wycombe
Bucks HP11 2QW
Tel.: 01494 437278
Helpline: 0845 305 2060
Website: www.coeliac.org.uk

There is also an office in Scotland:
Citibase Edinburgh
1 St Colme Street
Edinburgh EH3 6AA
Tel.: 0131 220 8342

Coeliac Society of Ireland
Carmichael House
4 North Brunswick Street
Dublin 7
Tel.: +353 1 872 1471
Website: www.coeliac.ie

Other UK health/autoimmune disease bodies

British Sjögren's Syndrome Association
Tel.: 0121 478 0222
Website: www.bssa.uk.net

British Society of Gastroenterology
Tel.: 020 7935 3150
Website: www.bsg.org.uk

British Thyroid Foundation
Tel.: 01423 709707
Website: www.btf-thyroid.org

Core (gut/liver health charity)
Tel.: 020 7486 0341
Website: www.corecharity.org.uk

Crohn's and Colitis UK (the working name of the National Association for Colitis and Crohn's Disease)
Tel.: 0845 130 2233 (information)
Website: www.nacc.org.uk

Diabetes UK
Tel.: 020 7424 1000
Website: www.diabetes.org.uk

The Gut Trust (IBS)
Tel.: 0872 300 4537 (helpline)
Website: www.thegutrust.org

Multiple Sclerosis Society
Tel.: 020 8438 0700
Website: www.mssociety.org.uk

NHS Choices (coeliac disease pages)
Website: www.nhs.uk/conditions/coeliac-disease

NICE (coeliac disease guidelines)
Website: www.nice.org.uk/CG86

National Osteoporosis Society
Tel.: 0845 4520 0230 (helpline)
Website: www.nos.org.uk

Eating out/travel guides

Celiac Travel: www.celiactravel.com

GlutenFreePassport: http://glutenfreepassport.com

Go Gluten Free Wheat Free: www.go-gluten-free-wheat-free.co.uk

Leave it Out: www.leaveitout.com

Special Gourmets: www.specialgourmets.com

Events

The Allergy & Gluten Free Show:
www.allergyshow.co.uk
The Free From Food Awards:
www.freefromfoodawards.co.uk
The Good Digestion Show: www.
thegooddigestionshow.co.uk

'Free from' food manufacturers

A number of these, the larger specialist 'free from' producers, will send welcome packs, vouchers and/ or samples if you get in touch or register online. All supermarkets, although not listed here, also have their own extensive 'free from' ranges, and can send or email lists of GF own-brand products. (*Denotes prescription supplier.)

Drossa UK Ltd*
Tel.: 020 3393 0859
Website: www.drossa.co.uk/www.
drossa.ltd.uk
Products: Pasta, gnocchi, flour/ bread/sweet mixes

General Dietary Ltd*
Tel.: 020 8336 2323
Website: www.generaldietary.com
Products: Ener-G pastas, breads, bakery sundries, cookies, communion wafers

Genius Gluten Free*
Tel.: 0845 874 4000
Website: www.geniusglutenfree.
com
Products: breads

GFF Direct*
Tel.: 01757 289200
Website: www.gffdirect.co.uk
Products: Feel-free pies, pasties and sausage rolls; Il Pana di Anna flour and pastas; Beiker breads, pastas and desserts; breakfast cereals, soups, drinks

Glebe Farm*
Tel.: 01487 773282
Website: www.glebe-flour.co.uk
Products: bread/flour/cake mixes

Gluten Free Foods Ltd*
Tel.: 020 8953 4444
Website: www.glutenfree-foods.
co.uk
Products: Barkat breads, pasta, flour mixes, snacks, biscuits, cakes, cereals

Hale & Hearty
Tel.: 020 7616 8427
Website: www.halenhearty.co.uk
Products: sweet and savoury mixes, cereals, pastas, snacks

Heron Quality Foods (Republic of Ireland)*****
Tel.: +353 0 233 9006/ +353 0 233 9960
Website: www.glutenfreedirect.com
Products: savoury and sweet mixes, cereals, biscuits

Innovative Solutions UK Ltd*
Tel.: 01706 746713/01706 341700
Website: www.innovative-solutions.
org.uk
Products: flours, baking ingredients

Juvela*
Tel.: 0800 783 1992
Website: www.juvela.co.uk
Products: breads, pasta, pizza bases, flour mixes, crackers, biscuits

Lifestyle Healthcare Ltd*
Tel.: 0845 270 1400
Website: www.gfdiet.com
Products: breads, savouries, pizza, sweet treats

Livwell*
Tel.: 0845 120 0038
Website: www.livwell.eu
Products: breads, pastries, cakes

MH Foods*
Tel.: 01322 337711
Website: www.mhfoods.net
Products: breads, mixes, crackers, cakes, sweet treats

Mrs Crimble's
Tel.: 08451 300 869
Website: www.mrscrimbles.com
Products: breads, mixes, crackers, cakes, sweet treats

Nutrition Point Ltd – Dietary Specials*
Tel.: 0800 954 1981
Website: www.dietaryspecials.co.uk
Products: breads, pastas, frozen meals, mixes, crackers, biscuits

Nutrition Point Ltd – Glutafin*
Tel.: 0800 988 2470
Website: www.glutafin.co.uk
Products: breads, flour mixes, pastas, crackers, biscuits

Nutrition Point Ltd – Trufree*
Tel.: 0800 954 1982 (UK); 1800 818 551 (ROI)
Website: www.trufree.co.uk
Products: crackers, biscuits

Orgran
Website: www.orgran.co.uk
Products: pasta, crispbreads, cereals, biscuits, soups, snacks, bread/flour mixes
Order via **Naturally Good Food***
(tel.: 01455 556878; website: www.naturallygoodfood.co.uk)

PGR Health Foods Ltd*
Tel.: 01992 581715
Website: www.pgrhealthfoods.co.uk
Products: Rizopia brown rice pastas

S.D.Parr & Co. Ltd*
Tel.: 01226 713044
Website: www.sdparr.co.uk
Products: Proceli breads from Spain, pastas, sweet bakery, ordered via the link <www.proceli.co.uk>.

Tobia Teff*
Tel.: 020 7328 2045
Website: www.tobiateff.co.uk
Products: teff flour and cereals

Wellfoods Ltd*
Tel.: 01226 381712
Website: www.wellfoods.co.uk
Products: breads, flour, pizza bases, muffins

Small/niche/online 'free from' producers

Against the Grain (cookies): www.againstthegrainfoods.com

Bia Nua (bakery ingredients): www.nianua.com

The Black Farmer (sausages): www.theblackfarmer.com

The Cake Crusader: www.thecakecrusader.co.uk

Celia's Kitchen (bakery): www.celiaskitchen.co.uk

Christine's Puddings (puddings): www.christinespuddings.co.uk

Conscious Food (snacks): www.consciousfood.co.uk

Cookroom (savouries, sweets): www.cookroom.co.uk

Delicious (Republic of Ireland; bakery): www.delicious.ie

Delicious Alchemy (bakery): www.deliciousalchemy.co.uk

Droppa & Droppa (various):
www.droppaanddroppa.com

Especially Delicious (bespoke cakes):
www.especiallydelicious.co.uk

Estrella Damm (beers):
www.estrelladamm.com/en

Foodamentalists (various):
www.foodamentalists.co.uk

G Free (sweet bakery):
www.gfree.co.uk

Glu-2-Go (batter mix, flavourings):
www.glu2go.co.uk

Gluten Free Goodies (sweet treats):
www.glutenfreegoodies.co.uk

Gluten Free Kitchen (bakery):
www.glutenfreefood.info

Green's Gluten Free Beers:
www.glutenfreebeers.co.uk

The Healthy Cake Company:
www.healthycakecompany.co.uk

Honeybuns (tarts, sweet treats):
www.honeybuns.co.uk

Intolerable Food Company
(various): www.intolerablefood.com

Isabel's Naturally Free From
(savouries):
www.brazilianflavours.net

JoJo's Cakes:
www.jojos-cakes.co.uk

Kelkin (Republic of Ireland; various): www.kelkin.ie

Kent & Fraser (biscuits, cakes):
www.kentandfraser.com

Lazy Day Foods (sweet treats):
www.lazydayfoods.com

Lovemore (bakery):
www.lovemore-freefromfoods.com

Morley's of Swanland (meat products):
www.glutenfreebutcher.co.uk

Roley's (teff bakery):
www.roleys.com

Sally's Sizzling Sausage Company:
www.sallyssizzlers.com

Steph's Free From Cakes:
www.stephsfreefromcakes.co.uk

Tilquhillie Fine Foods (GF oats):
www.tilquhilliefinefoods.com

Online shops

Dietary Needs Direct: www.dietaryneedsdirect.co.uk

Ecodirect Ltd (Republic of Ireland): www.ecodirect.ie

FreeFoods.co.uk: www.freefoods.co.uk

Gluten Free Shop Ltd: www.gluten-freeshop.co.uk

Simply Free: www.simply-free.co.uk

WheatandDairyFree.com: www.wheatanddairyfree.com

Miscellaneous websites

Coeliac Youth of Europe: http://cye.freehostia.com

Coeliac Coach (Republic of Ireland): www.coeliaccoach.com

FoodsYouCan ('free from' food info): www.foodsyoucan.co.uk

Gluten Free Cooking for Kids: www.glutenfree4kids.com

Social networking

A small selection of active online accounts and forums, which are a good source of coeliac news, tips, recipes, research and debate.

Facebook
Coeliac Disease – not just a food preference: www.facebook.com/coeliac

Coeliac London: www.facebook.com/coeliaclondon

Coeliac UK: www.facebook.com/CoeliacUK

Coeliac Society of Ireland: www.facebook.com/CoeliacSocIreland

Gluten-free Foodies: www.facebook.com/glutenfreefoodies

Twitter
Hashtags regularly used in coeliac-related tweets include, among others, #coeliac#celiac#glutenfree #gfree.

Author, Alex Gazzola: www.twitter.com/HealthJourno

Coeliac UK: www.twitter.com/coeliac_uk

FoodsMatter.com: www.twitter.com/foodsmatter

Gluten Free Media: www.twitter.com/GlutenFreeMedia

Chat forums
Some of the other organizations mentioned in this Useful addresses section have chat forums too.

The Gluten Free Message Board: http://members2.boardhost.com/glutenfree

Foodreactions.org: www.foodreactions.org/forum

North American coeliac organizations

American Celiac Disease Alliance
Tel.: +1-703-622-3331; website: www.americanceliac.org

Canadian Celiac Association
Tel.: +1-905-507-6208; website: www.celiac.ca

Celiac Disease Foundation
Tel.: +1-818-990-2354; website: www.celiac.org

Celiac Sprue Association
Tel.: +1-877-272-4272; website: www.csaceliacs.org

Gluten Intolerance Group of North America
Tel.: +1-253-833-6655; website: www.gluten.net

National Foundation for Celiac Awareness
Tel.: +1-215-325-1306; website: www.celiaccentral.org

US coeliac disease centres

The University of Chicago Celiac Disease Center: www.celiacdisease.net

Columbia University Celiac Disease Center: www.celiacdiseasecenter.columbia.edu

University of Maryland Center for Celiac Research: www.celiaccenter.org

Other international coeliac societies

Non-anglophone nations offering English-language sections and/or advice to visitors on their sites are marked with an asterisk.

Europe
Österreichische Arbeitsgemeinschaft Zöliakie (Austria): www.zoeliakie.or.at

Vlaamse Coeliakie Vereniging (Belgium – Flemish-speaking): vcv.coeliakie.be*

Société Belge de la Coeliaquie (Belgium – French-speaking): www.sbc-asbl.be*

Hrvatsko Društvo za Celijakiju (Croatia): www.celijakija.hr*

Společnost pro bezlepkovou dietu (Czech Republic): http://celiak.cz/en*

Dansk Cøliaki Forening (Denmark): www.coeliaki.dk

Keliakialiitto (Finland): www.keliakialiitto.fi*

Association Française des Intolérants au Gluten (France): www.afdiag.org

Deutsche Zöliakie Gesellschaft (Germany): www.dzg-online.de*

Greek Coeliac Society: www.koiliokaki.com*

Lisztérzékenyek Érdekképviseletének Országos Egyesülete (Hungary): www.coeliac.hu/tiki-index.php

Associazione Italiana Celiachia (Italy): www.celiachia.it*

Nederlandse Coeliakie Vereniging (Netherlands): www.glutenvrij.nl*

Norsk Cøliakiforening (Norway): www.ncf.no*

Polskie Stowarzyszenie Osøb z Celiakia I Na Diecie Bezglutenowej (Poland): www.celiakia.org.pl

Associação Portuguesa de Celíacos (Portugal): www.celiacos.org.pt

Celiakia (Slovakia): www.celiakia.sk

Slovensko Drustvo za Celiakijo (Slovenia): www.drustvo-celiakija.si

Federación de Asociaciones de Celíacos de España (Spain): www.celiacos.org*

Svenska Celiakiförbundet (Sweden): www.celiaki.se*

IC Zöliakie der Deutschen Schweiz (Switzerland): www.zoeliakie.ch

Asia and Oceania
The Coeliac Society of Australia: www.coeliacsociety.com.au

The Israeli Celiac Association: www.celiac.org.il*

Coeliac New Zealand: www.coeliac.co.nz

Pakistani Celiac Society: www.celiac.com.pk*

Çölyakla Yaşam Derneği (Turkey): www.colyak.org.tr

Index